THE GOOD
NUTRITION GUIDE

THE GOOD
NUTRITION GUIDE

Published by the Ethical Marketing Group

First edition published 2008 by The Ethical Marketing Group

The Ethical Company Organisation
105 Westbourne Grove, London W2 4UW
www.ethical-company-organisation.org

© Ethical Company Organisation 2008

Telephone: 0845 257 6818

Research and Editorial Director - William Sankey
Publishing and Accreditation Director - Kat Alexander
Written and Edited by Sarah Edwards

ISBN 978-0-9552907-2-5

Distributed by Central Books (Orders @ centralbooks.com 0845 458 9911)
Sales enquires to Signature Books (sales@signaturebooks.co.uk 01904 633633)

Legal Disclaimer
The Good Nutrition Guide aims to provide an independent and authoritative list of mainstream brands and companies according to research executed by The Ethical Company Organisation. While every reasonable care is taken to ensure the accuracy of the information in The Good Nutrition Guide, neither the publisher, the printers nor any distributor is responsible for errors or omissions. Check the 'nutrition facts' on product labels for the very latest nutritional information as products change ingredients frequently.

Contents

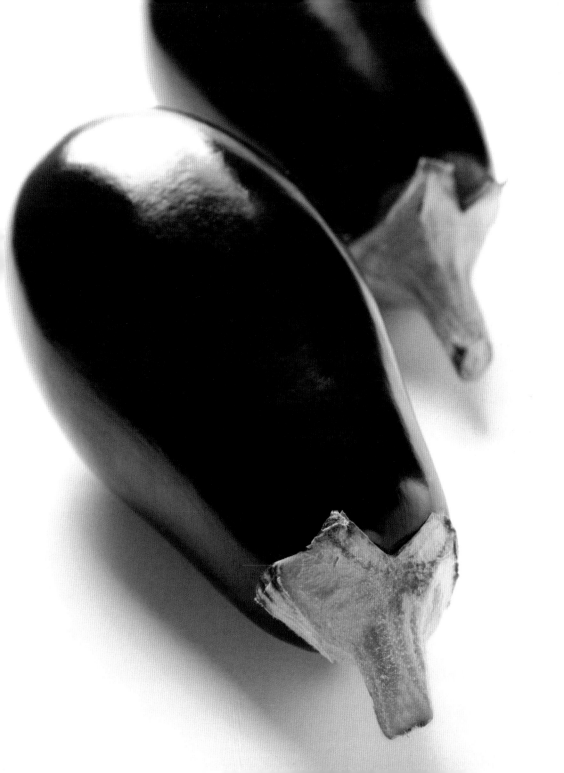

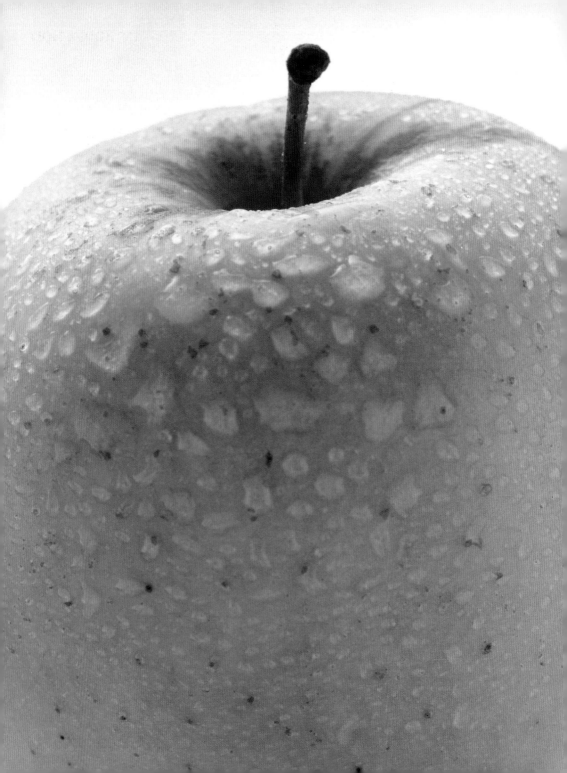

Foreword

In reality, improving diet isn't only about fresh fruit and vegetables - it is also about choosing healthier brands over those packed with damaging sugar, salt, fat and additives. The link between diet and a range of life-threatening conditions such as obesity, heart disease, high blood pressure, cancer and diabetes is clear.

Working with the Food Standards Agency official guidelines on sugar, fat, salt and fibre, *The Good Nutrition Guide* at last reveals the true health rankings of UK food brands. Hundreds of famous food products (from Heniz to Hob Nobs) are analysed and compared in detail.

The Good Nutrition Guide also puts these ground-breaking league tables into context, providing pages of healthy eating information and good nutrition advice.

The proven links between good nutrition, vitality, health and happiness are being strengthened with every study. *The Good Nutrition Guide* provides shockingly clear information - and shows why good nutrition starts with knowing exactly which are the heroes and villains of the supermarket shelves!

William Sankey
Research Director
The Ethical Company Organisation

Why Choose Good Nutrition?

Most of us don't bother to check the labels when we're shopping for groceries: we assume that there is little difference between the foods we buy at the supermarket. Such wishful thinking is not good for us, or our bodies – as this book will show. In reality, there is often a big nutritional difference between food choices. Take, for example, the ready-made lasagnes that contain more than a day's recommended intake of salt, breakfast cereals made with generous helpings of vegetable oil and sugary yoghurts that offer the "flavour" of an ingredient without a hint of the real thing.

More and more processed foods are being uncovered as "HFSS"; high in fat, salt and sugar. HFSS foods are associated with weight gain and are a major cause of obesity in Britain. The proportion of men in England who were classified as obese rose from 13 per cent to 23 per cent between 1993 and 2004, and the Department of Health predicts that in England alone 12 million adults and one million children will be obese by 2010. Deficiency diseases such as scurvy may have virtually disappeared from Britain, but other conditions have taken their place: overnutrition, rather than undernutrition, is now common.

The consequences of this collective weight gain are far reaching, but the greatest concern should be for the nation's physical well-being. Carrying excess weight has long been associated with health problems, but the full extent of the risks are only just being uncovered. So severe are the implications of obesity that some doctors now describe it as a disease in its own right. Some of the most widespread chronic diseases in the UK are now believed to have direct links to diet:

CARDIOVASCULAR DISEASE

Cardiovascular disease kills one in three people in the UK and is the biggest cause of death in the US and most of Europe.

It affects the heart and surrounding arteries, and involves a process called atherosclerosis, in which fatty deposits from cholesterol and other substances build up in the arteries. These deposits, called plaque, narrow the arteries and reduce blood flow. If they break free they can cause a heart attack or stroke. Eating saturated and hydrogenated (trans) fats – often found in processed cakes, biscuits and crisps – increases the levels of LDL cholesterol in the blood, and can contribute to atherosclerosis and the development of cardiovascular disease in later life. Limiting your consumption of these fats, and eating more "good" HDL cholesterol from oily fish, nuts and seeds, can protect against the harmful effects of LDL cholesterol.

HIGH BLOOD PRESSURE

High blood pressure (hypertension) is a "silent killer"; a potentially deadly condition that you may not even know you have. It affects one third of people in England, and is often associated with eating too much salt, taking too little exercise, being overweight and drinking too much alcohol. Having high blood pressure makes you three times more likely to develop heart disease, and increases your risk of suffering a stroke. Many people with high blood pressure have no symptoms, so it is crucial to be aware of the causes and to know if you are likely to be at risk.

TYPE 2 DIABETES

Type 2 used to be referred to as "adult-onset" diabetes, but the number of young people being diagnosed with the condition has increased rapidly over the last decade. Unlike Type 1 diabetes, this form of the disease is associated with lifestyle. Eating too much sugary food alone will not cause diabetes, but it will greatly increase the risk factors in those who are genetically predisposed to the condition: 80 per cent of patients treated for Type 2 diabetes are overweight.

Type 2 diabetes occurs when the body builds up resistance to insulin, the hormone that regulates glucose levels in the blood. In people with diabetes, the body's diminished response to insulin means that the cells do not properly absorb glucose. The disease can usually be managed using a combination of diet, exercise and weight loss, but if left untreated it can cause serious problems including kidney failure and blindness. Maintaining a balanced diet and a healthy weight is one way of reducing your risk of developing this condition.

CANCER

It is now thought that one third of cancers are related to diet. According to Cancer Research UK, consumption of alcohol can increase the risk of liver, breast and bowel cancer, particularly amongst people who also smoke. The organisation lists links between red meat and bowel cancer, and a possible association between salt and stomach cancer. A diet high in fibre, high in fruit and vegetables and low in fat can help reduce many of the risks.

Eating the wrong foods could make you more likely to develop these diseases, but while a balanced diet can help to guard against problems in the future, good nutrition is not just about preventative action. In combination with an active lifestyle, eating the right food is crucial for everyday health.

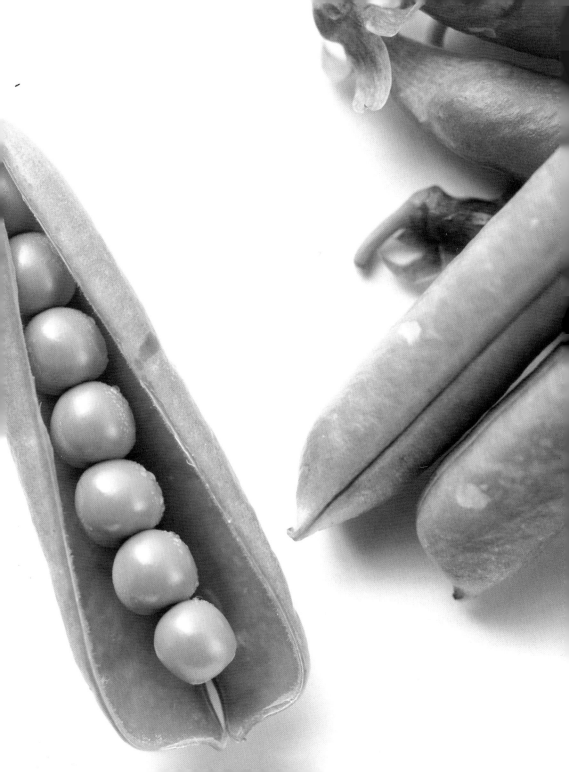

What is Good Nutrition?

Good nutrition is about understanding why you eat the foods you eat. It is about empowering consumers to make an informed choice about each and every product they buy. And, most of all, it is about eating well.

Of all the factors affecting our day-to-day health, nutrition should be one of the easiest to modify. But with the average supermarket stocking over 26,000 lines it is not always easy to know where to begin. *The Good Nutrition Guide* will provide you with that starting point. Part One introduces the key principles of nutrition, featuring up-to-date guidance from leading independent groups and government bodies. It shows how to put these principles into practice, and provides tips on "label watching" and making the healthiest choices at the shops.

Part Two introduces the Ethical Company Organisation's unique, impartial research into the nutritional value of processed goods. Using the Food Standards Agency's established criteria for HFSS foods, it has rated hundreds of products for their nutrient content, allowing you to make instant comparisons between the biggest brand names on the shelf. How do Kellogg's cereals compare to Nestlé's? Are Walkers crisps higher or lower in fat than Pringles? Which cheeses are most suitable for someone on a low salt diet? The second half of this book will reveal all.

The Good Nutrition Guide shows you how to make positive choices about your food purchases. By applying its nutrition tables to the products you most frequently buy, you will be able to see the true value of the foods you eat. If you want to look after your health and reduce your chances of becoming overweight or developing high blood pressure or high cholesterol, you need to know what's in your food, from the biggest food groups to the smallest additives. Improving your diet means being informed and pro-active: by buying this book you have taken the first step towards good nutrition.

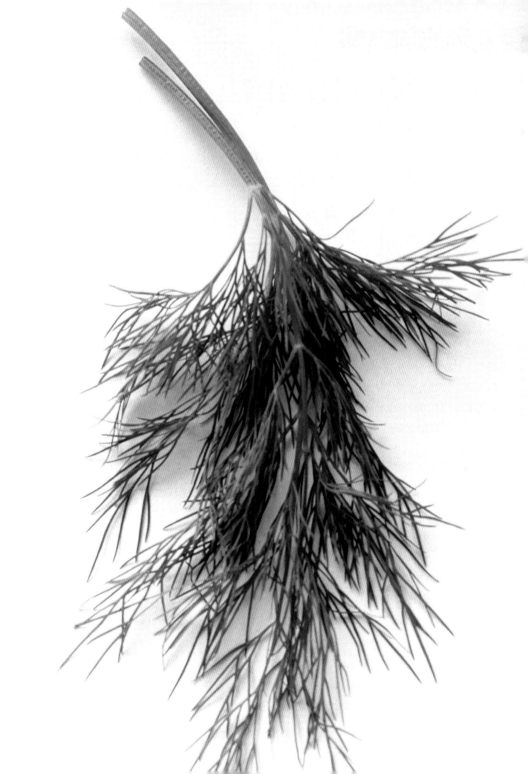

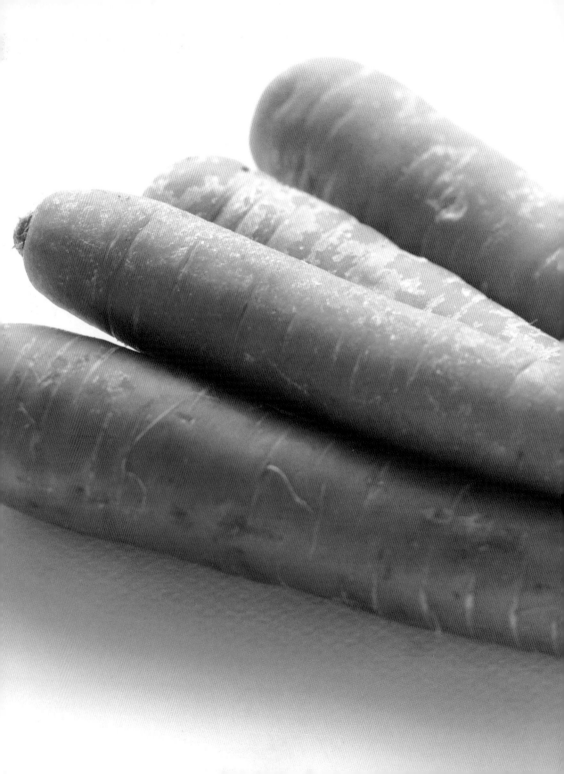

PRINCIPLES OF GOOD NUTRITION

KNOW YOUR NUTRIENTS •
GET YOUR BALANCE •

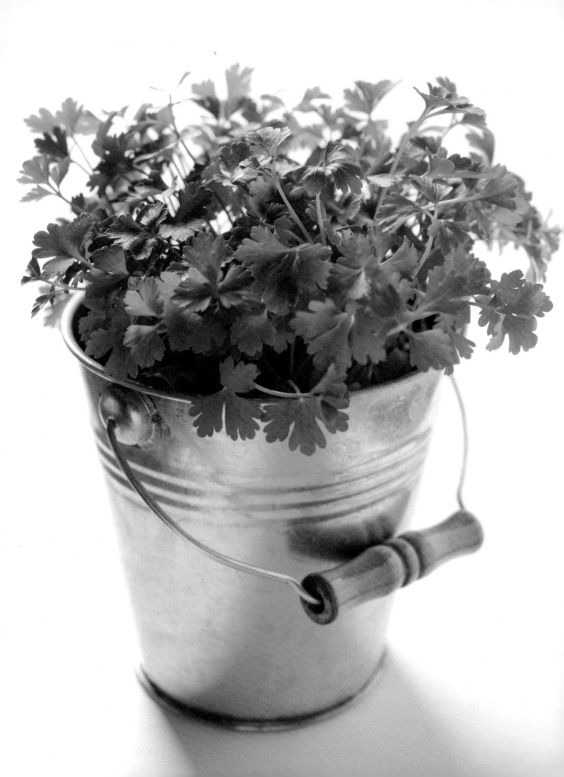

Know Your Nutrients

Nutrients are the stuff of life. They are the substances at the heart of our physiology. Taken into the body every time we eat or drink, they have an influence at all levels of our existence, and are involved in everything from the tiniest cellular changes to the biggest chemical reactions. By providing us with energy they keep us going on a day-to-day basis, as well as enabling us to grow, survive and reproduce. Without them, we could not exist.

Nutrients provide us with the raw materials we need to keep the cells, organs and organ systems in the body working in harmony. The complex process of balancing and regulating these internal systems is called homeostasis, and is influenced by our outside environment including the temperature, the composition of the air and the time of day. All the nutrients we take in have an influence on these internal systems. While most people in wealthy countries now have access to all the nourishment they need, getting the nutrient balance right can still be difficult for one simple reason: we don't just eat nutrients, we eat food.

All foods contain nutrients, but they appear in different levels according to the type of food and how it has been prepared.

For example, a cooked carrot may have fewer vitamins than a raw one, but the chances are it will still contain more than a carrot cake. Nutrients are grouped into a number of different categories, which are often known as the five major food groups: proteins, carbohydrates, fats, fibre and vitamins/minerals.

Although all of these nutrient types are indispensable, some of them – such as vitamins – are required in lower levels than others. Recommended daily amounts are now available for all the major food groups, providing guidance on the optimum intakes for the average adult. To understand why these figures have been given, and how to translate them into a balanced diet, we need to know what effect each nutrient group has on the body. These effects form the basis of the principles of good nutrition.

1) PROTEIN

Proteins are best known for their role in growth and repair, but they also have dozens of other uses within the body. Some act as catalysts, helping to speed up the chemical reactions that take place in the cells. Others play a part in the immune system, or are used as transporters and messengers in the blood. It is now thought that there are hundreds of thousands of proteins in the human body – more than there are genes in our DNA. The existence of such vast numbers of proteins is explained in the way they are made.

An individual protein is made up of many amino acids, which join together through connections called peptide bonds to form polypeptides. There may be up to 500 amino acids in one polypeptide. The number of amino acids in a polypeptide chain and the sequence in which they bond determines what kind of protein they produce. Just 20 types of amino acid are found in the proteins we eat, but these can combine to form hundreds of different proteins, each with a different shape and function.

When a protein is eaten, the body breaks it down into its constituent amino acids. These can then be used individually or rearranged to form new proteins. Although the body can make some amino acids, others have to be obtained from food. The ones that we cannot make ourselves are known as "essential amino acids", and it is crucial that we include them in our diet. For human adults, there are eight essential amino acids: leucine, isoleucine, valine, threonine, methionine, phenylalanine, tryptophan and lysine.

The more of these essential amino acids are found in a food, the higher its biological value or "quality". A high quality protein will provide essential and non-essential amino acids in the proportions that the body needs. Proteins from animals (such as meat, fish and dairy products) are of higher quality than proteins from plants (such as vegetables, pulses and seeds). This is why vegetarians are often advised to use "protein combining" to make sure that the limitations of one type of protein are compensated for by another. However, recent thinking on the subject suggests that this may not be necessary, as a balanced diet will provide reasonable amounts of all the essential amino acids.

In fact, the majority of us may be eating significantly more protein than we actually need. While the Food Standards Agency's guidelines say that men need 44–55g of protein a day, and women need 36–45g, the British Nutrition Foundation estimates that the average daily intake is 88g for men and 64g for women. In Britain, two thirds of our protein intake is from meat and dairy products. As proteins should only contribute to 15 per cent of our daily calorie intake, these foods (which are also high in fat) should be eaten in moderation.

Good animal sources of protein include lean meat, poultry, eggs and fish. Cheese, milk and yoghurt are good dairy sources, although these should be limited to two or three servings per day. Pulses (such as lentils and beans) are a particularly healthy plant source, as are tofu and other products made from soya. 100g of tofu contains almost as much protein as a chicken breast. Protein is also found in bread and cereals, brown rice, nuts and seeds.

As so many of our staple foods contain protein, if you eat a balanced diet containing plenty of pulses and grains alongside moderate servings of animal and diary products, you will be getting plenty of this nutrient, and a good supply of the essential amino acids.

2) CARBOHYDRATE

Carbohydrates are our main source of energy, and can be used directly as fuel or stored as glycogen within the muscles and liver. "Blood sugar" is carbohydrate that has been broken down into glucose and is ready to be transported to the cells, where it will be needed for chemical reactions and other mechanisms. Although providing energy is by far their biggest function, carbohydrates are also involved in processes such as blood clotting and fertilisation, and are an important part of some of the body's more complex proteins.

There are three main groups of carbohydrates. Monosaccharides are single molecules such as glucose and fructose. Disaccharides are made from two monosaccharides joined together; for example, glucose and fructose combine to form sucrose, commonly known as table sugar. Polysaccharides (such as starch) are long chains, and may be made from many thousands of single glucose molecules. When a polysaccharide carbohydrate is digested, it is separated back into its constituent parts and these glucose molecules are released.

In nutritional terms, carbohydrates are divided into two categories, complex and simple. It is these that are included on food labels as "Carbohydrates" and "Carbohydrates (of which sugars)". Complex carbohydrates are polysaccharides or "starchy" foods such as potatoes and pasta. Simple carbohydrates are sugars, including those found naturally in fruits, vegetables and milk, and those used as sweeteners such as honey.

Although some popular diets advocate "cutting down the carbs", complex carbohydrates are a healthy option. With 1 gram of carbohydrate providing 3.75kcal (16kj) of energy – half as much as a gram of fat – they are not as calorie-laden as many people think. It is recommended that carbohydrates should make up about 50 per cent of our daily calorie intake. Where we should be cutting down is the added sugars that appear in sweetened products such as cakes and biscuits. The typical British diet obtains more energy than it should from these simple carbohydrates.

The figure for "Carbohydrates (of which sugars)" does not tell you how much comes from fruit or milk sugars and how much has been added. As a general guideline, the Food Standards Agency states that 10g sugars or more per 100g is a lot of sugar and 2g sugars or less per 100g is a little sugar. In between 2g and 10g per 100g is a moderate amount. The recommended daily allowance for carbohydrates is 230g, of which 90g can be sugars. Added sugars are not always easy to identify from the nutrition label, as they tend to be concealed within the ingredients list. Sugars to watch out for include glucose, maltose, honey and corn syrup.

For men, the average daily intake of carbohydrate is 275g. For women it is 203g. Almost half of this figure comes from cereal and cereal products, including bread, followed by 12 per cent from potatoes and potato snacks. The easiest way to ensure we are eating enough complex carbohydrates is to base our meals around them, for example by combining pasta and sauce. Starchy foods include bread (tortillas, pitta breads and chapattis as well as ordinary loaves), potatoes and sweet potatoes, squash, wholegrain breakfast cereals, lentils, beans, couscous and oats.

Fruits and vegetables are nutritious

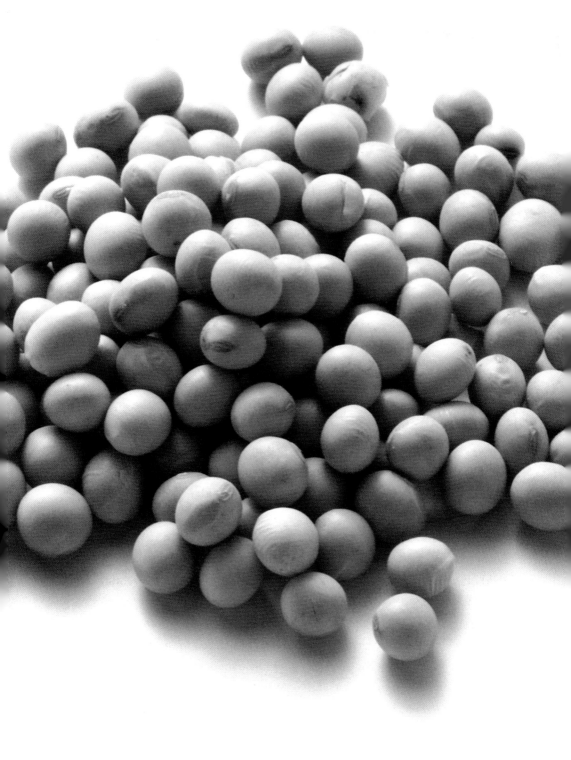

sources of carbohydrate, and should be included in the diet as part of your five-a-day. They are also a good source of a particular type of carbohydrate called fibre, which will be looked at in more detail later in the chapter. Satisfy a sweet tooth with fresh fruit rather than foods containing added sugars, and eat plenty of complex carbohydrates to get the most from this energy-rich nutrient.

3) FAT

Although fat has something of a bad reputation, the body could not do without it. As well as being a much more concentrated energy source than either protein or carbohydrate, providing 9kcal (37kj) of energy per gram, it is also used to carry soluble vitamins in the blood. The fats we eat are either used immediately for energy or stored in adipose tissue. This is found around the major organs (where it acts as a protective barrier), and as an insulating layer under the skin. If more fat is taken in than the body can use up as energy, the adipose tissue accumulates, making a person overweight.

When fat is digested, its two components, fatty acids and glycerol, are released into the blood. Glycerol is taken to the liver where it is converted into glucose to be used – like the glucose from carbohydrate – as fuel in the body's cells. Fatty acids are also a source of fuel, or may be used in other structural roles. The body can make all but two of the fatty acids it needs. Alpha linolenic acid and linoleic acid belong to the group of omega-3 and 6 fats, and must be found in the diet. Good sources include oily fish and foods produced by animals fed an omega-3 enriched diet.

There are three main types of fat in the human diet, and they are named according to the structure of their fatty acid molecules. All fatty acids are made from chains of carbon atoms, which are attached to different numbers of hydrogen atoms. A saturated fatty acid is one that is attached to the maximum possible number of hydrogen atoms; an unsaturated fatty acid has room for more. In an unsaturated fat, the space where the hydrogen atom would be is replaced with a double bond: a monounsaturated fat has one of these spaces and one double bond, while a polyunsaturated fat has many.

The significance of this structure is the role it is thought to play in the properties of the fat. Saturated fats (such as those found in butter, hard cheeses, meat pies and cakes) increase the level of cholesterol in the blood, which leads to a greater risk of heart disease. Unsaturated fats, on the other hand, can help reduce the level of cholesterol in the blood. These are found in oily fish, nuts and seeds, olive oil and avocados.

However, one type of polyunsaturated fat, trans fat, is associated with increased cholesterol. Trans fats are found naturally in some meat and dairy products, and are also made during hydrogenation, a process used in the production of margarine. They appear in many fast foods and baked goods such as cakes. Although trans fats have been the subject of much controversy, the FSA estimates that the average person consumes only half the recommended maximum each day.

In general, we should be reducing our intake of fat, particularly saturated fats. The guideline daily amount is 70g total fats, with 20g of this being saturates. On the nutrition label, 20g total fat and 5g saturated fat or more per 100g is high; 3g total fat and 1g saturated fat per 100g is low. Ways of reducing saturated fats in the diet include choosing low fat versions of

products such as milk and cheese. Cutting the fat and skin from meats and grilling or baking foods rather than frying and roasting them will also help.

Even though fat provides large quantities of energy, it is less satiating than protein and carbohydrate, meaning it doesn't produce the same feeling of being full. Less than a third of our energy intake should be from fat. Although this nutrient has a vital role in the body, too much of it is not a good thing.

4) FIBRE

While other nutrients such as fat and protein have to be broken down before they can be used within the body, fibre's unique quality is that it cannot be fully digested. Instead it forms the "roughage" or "bulk" that the digestive system needs to keep foods and their by-products moving through the intestines. It also helps to regulate the levels of sugar in the blood, which is an important part of treatment for people with diet-managed diabetes.

Fibre helps to guard against bowel disorders such as Crohn's disease and inflammation, as well as preventing constipation. Low fibre intake is associated with colon cancer, although it is not yet known if an increased intake has a protective effect. However, a diet that is high in fibre is also likely to be lower in the foods that cause an increased risk of cardiovascular disease, high cholesterol and obesity, making this a particularly important nutrient within the diet as a whole.

All fibre comes from plants, and the term "dietary fibre" is used to indicate any fibrous plant material that is not digested by the body. Dietary fibre can be categorised into two main types: soluble and insoluble. Insoluble fibre is resistant to the enzymes secreted by the digestive system, so it passes along the gut without being broken down. Soluble fibre is fibre that can be partially digested. While we cannot fully digest fibre ourselves, the bacteria that live in our guts can act upon both types. These microorganisms ferment or partially ferment the fibre to release gas and fatty acids that we can use as energy. This is why gut bacteria (varieties of which are sold commercially in "probiotic" products) are important to intestinal health.

Most foods contain a combination of insoluble and soluble fibres in varying proportions, so it is important to eat a variety of vegetable products to ensure you are getting enough of both. Soluble fibre can help reduce cholesterol, making it a crucial part of a healthy diet. Good sources of soluble fibre include oats (for example in the form of muesli or porridge) and pulses such as beans and lentils. Insoluble fibre is found in fruit and vegetables, brown rice and wholegrain foods such as granary bread.

In Britain, most people don't have enough fibre in their diet. Vegetarians and vegans tend to eat more than meat-eaters because their meals are based largely on vegetables and pulses. The average intake is 12g per day, which is less than the recommended level of 18g. At the moment there is some disagreement over which plant substances count as dietary fibre, so if the classification changes this recommended figure may actually be higher.

A high fibre food is one that contains 6g of fibre or more per 100g. The Food Standards Agency advises that to be labelled as a "source" of fibre a food must contain 3g or more per 100g. If a product has not had fibre added but is a naturally good source it can be described as "a high fibre food". Some people are discouraged from increasing their fibre intake by the possibility of excess wind or bloating, but these symptoms should soon diminish as the bacteria in the gut adapt. Drinking more water may alleviate the problem by helping the fibre to move more easily through the gut.

The main sources of fibre in the average diet are bread and breakfast cereals, but fresh fruit and vegetables, pulses, oats, beans and unrefined (wholemeal) carbohydrates are also high in this nutrient, and provide a good basis for a healthy fibre intake.

5) SALT

Salt is the common name for a compound called sodium chloride. The body needs the sodium from sodium chloride to help it regulate the amount of water in the blood. Sodium is also used in the transmission of electrical signals in the nerves, and aids the absorption of nutrients from the gut. Like other minerals such as iron (which will be looked at in more detail later in this chapter), only very small quantities of salt are required.

In Britain, 85 per cent of men and 69 per cent of women eat too much salt.

This is particularly worrying because salt has been linked to high blood pressure. A high sodium intake causes the body to retain more water, which increases the amount of fluid in the blood vessels. Over time, the raised pressure cause by this increase in fluid can damage the vessel walls, leading to a higher risk of cardiovascular problems. According to the Department of Health, people with high blood pressure are three times more likely to suffer from heart attack and stroke than those without. One third of Britons have high blood pressure.

On average, we eat 9.5g of salt per day, which is 60 per cent more than the recommended level. As over three quarters of the salt we eat is "hidden" – included in processed foods such as bread, soups and even sweet products such as biscuits – many of us may not realise that we are exceeding our recommended daily intake, even if we don't add salt to our foods at home. The maximum amount of salt we should be eating per day is 6g, or about a teaspoon.

The Food Standards Agency is campaigning for better labelling of salt on processed products so that consumers know exactly what they are eating. At the moment most manufacturers list sodium, rather than salt, which may lead people to believe they are consuming less salt than they actually are. The FSA's guidelines state that 0.6g sodium or more per 100g is "a lot", and 0.1g sodium or less per 100g is "a little". The maximum recommended daily amount for sodium is 2.5g. To work out the amount of salt from the figure in grams for sodium, multiply it by 2.5.

Foods that may be high in added salt include breakfast cereals, baked beans, cook-in sauces, condiments such as tomato ketchup and ready meals. Some ready meals contain almost a whole day's salt intake in one portion, which may be easy to miss if the nutrient levels are given per 100g rather than per serving. Anchovies, bacon, hard cheese, olives, sausages, soy sauce, stock cubes and yeast spreads are all high salt foods. Small quantities of salt are naturally present in most raw foods.

It is possible to reduce your salt intake by adding less, or no, salt to foods at home. Avoiding salty crisps, nuts and snacks can help, as can choosing low-salt versions of products such as biscuits, cheese and ready meals. Even tinned

vegetables may contain this nutrient as a preservative or flavour enhancer, so pick the ones that are labelled "no added salt". The taste buds react quickly to changes in diet, so a palate that is used to salty foods will soon adjust to the lower levels.

A small amount of salt is essential for good health, but until changes are made within the food industry to limit the amount found in processed products, it is up to us to ensure we are not getting too much.

6) VITAMINS AND MINERALS

Vitamins and minerals are nutrients that are required in very small quantities (usually measured in micrograms, µg, or milligrams, mg) for the body to function. Almost all of these are substances that cannot be synthesised internally, meaning that they must be obtained from the diet. The amount of vitamins and minerals needed varies according to age and sex, and the Department of Health publishes Dietary Reference Values giving guidelines and recommended intakes for each one (www.dh.gov.uk). A balanced and varied diet should provide all the vitamins and minerals we need, but in some cases – such as for people with anaemia – supplementation is necessary.

VITAMINS

Vitamin deficiency is no longer a major health problem in the UK, but eating a restrictive or limited diet or one low in fresh produce can reduce the number of vitamins consumed. With the exception of some B vitamins and vitamin D, which can be produced when the skin is exposed to sunlight, all of these nutrients need to be found in the foods we eat. Overcooking food, for example by boiling vegetables, can destroy their vitamin content; steaming is often a better option. Many foods are now fortified with the essential vitamins.

Below is a list of major vitamins, their uses in the body and good sources to include in the diet.

Vitamin A

Vitamin A is needed for growth and differentiation of cells, healthy skin and the maintenance of eyesight. Good sources are liver and dairy foods including whole milk and cheese, leafy green vegetables, carrots and orange coloured fruits such as apricots.

B Vitamins

There are many B vitamins, of which B6 and B12 – which are needed to maintain the levels of homocysteine in the blood – are perhaps most widely known. Raised homocysteine has been linked with cardiovascular disease. B12 is only found in animal products, while B6 also occurs in wholegrains and vegetables.

Vitamin C

Vitamin C has a role in keeping blood vessels working, and is involved in the maintenance of skin and bone. Smokers use up the useful substances in vitamin C more quickly, so need to make sure they get plenty of it in the diet. It can be found in fruits and vegetables, including potatoes, as well as dairy products.

Vitamin D

This vitamin is used for cell division and in the promotion of bone structure. The body can produce vitamin D, but the diet is another important source. All margarines in the UK are fortified with vitamin D, and it also appears in eggs and oily fish.

Vitamin K

Used for blood clotting and bone structure, vitamin K can be found in various plant and animal sources including green leafy vegetables and meat. We also make small quantities of it ourselves in the intestine.

Folate

Folate or folic acid is needed for cell division, and is particularly important in pregnancy because of its role in the development of the embryo. Foods such as breakfast cereals are now fortified with folic acid, although it also appears naturally in brown rice, green vegetables, bananas and chickpeas.

MINERALS

Although mineral deficiency is relatively rare in the UK, some sections of the population, particularly adolescents, are at risk of not getting enough iron, calcium and trace elements such as zinc. However, in most cases the levels are not low enough to cause any adverse symptoms.

Even though they are required in only tiny amounts, minerals play a vital part in major processes such as bone formation and controlling the levels of fluid in the body. The essential minerals, which also include salt, are:

Calcium

Calcium is important for strong bones and teeth, particularly in children and teenagers as their skeletons are still developing. Dairy products such as milk and cheese are rich in calcium, and it can also be found in soya beans, green vegetables such as broccoli and bread made with fortified flour.

Iron

The body needs iron to help make red blood cells, which it uses to carry oxygen in the blood. Red meats are particularly good sources of iron, but it also occurs in dried fruits, beans, nuts and green leafy vegetables. The tannins in tea can reduce the amount of iron absorbed in digestion, while vitamin C is thought to have a positive effect on its uptake.

Magnesium

Magnesium is used in the conversion of food into energy. It also has a role in the function of muscle. This nutrient is especially present in nuts and green leafy vegetables.

Phosphorus

This is needed to maintain the structure of bones and teeth, and appears in meat and dairy products, oats and bread.

Potassium

Helps to control body fluid levels. Bananas are a good source, as are other vegetables, pulses and poultry.

Sulphur

This is involved in the production of cartilage. It is used as a preservative and appears naturally in most foods.

Alongside the essential minerals, trace elements are needed in even smaller quantities. They fulfil a variety of functions and are found in many different foods including animal products, cereals, vegetables and nuts. Trace elements include copper, iodine, selenium, zinc and many more. Eating a balanced diet that incorporates these foods will ensure you are getting enough.

7) WATER

Water is not traditionally classified as a nutrient, but it has been included here because it is a vitally important constituent of a balanced diet. It helps us to regulate our body temperature, enables chemical reactions to take place in the cells, lubricates our joints, helps us to swallow, and facilitates the transport of nutrients in the blood. Lack of this vital liquid is fatal.

Water, or H_2O, consists of two hydrogen atoms and an oxygen atom, and is one of the most abundant compounds on the planet. As well as a wide range of natural, social and industrial uses it is also a vital component of our diet, as a liquid for drinking and a binding ingredient in cooking. In processed foods, water only appears on the label if it makes up more than 5 per cent of the finished product.

Two thirds of our body weight is water, and losing just 2 per cent of this can put us at risk of dehydration. We lose water naturally through the production of urine, a process the body uses to excrete the toxic by-products of digestion. Water is also lost through evaporation from the tongue and in sweat. Symptoms of mild dehydration include headaches and tiredness, lack of concentration and confusion – the urine is visibly darker in colour because less water is being lost in this way.

The amount of water we need varies according to age, diet and lifestyle, and the climate we live in. The Food Standards Agency recommends an average daily water intake of six to eight glasses (approximately 1.5 litres) per day in Britain. This can take the form of pure water, hot drinks including tea and coffee, plus squash or fruit juice. Water contains no calories, and is a better choice for dental health than sugary juices and soft drinks.

Caffeinated drinks such as coffee have a slight diuretic effect, meaning that they cause an increase in the amount of urine produced. This response is negligible in comparison to the quantity of fluid taken in from the drink, but caffeinated beverages should not be the only source of water in the diet. Alcohol has a more marked effect, and strong drinks such as wine and spirits can be particularly dehydrating. Drinking water alongside alcohol can help to prevent dehydration, the main cause of hangovers.

As well as drinking, one third of our water intake comes from food, particularly fruit and vegetables. Dairy products are also a dietary source, but the small amount of water provided from these cannot take the place of a regular fluid intake. The feeling of thirst is a sign that the body is already lacking in water, so it is best to replace any lost fluids before you become too thirsty. This is particularly important in hot weather or following periods of exercise.

There is very little nutritional difference between tap and bottled water. Some commercial waters may contain extra minerals, but these should already be provided by a balanced diet. Tap water can be either hard or soft. Hard waters are those that contain dissolved minerals, particularly calcium and magnesium, and cause "furring" on kettles and other appliances. They are not thought to have any adverse affect on health, and some studies have suggested that they might even be beneficial.

PRINCIPLES OF GOOD NUTRITION

So far we have seen what the major nutrients are and what roles they play in keeping us active and healthy. This information can be summarised in the following principles of good nutrition:

1) Nutrients are nourishing substances that are obtained from food. All living creatures require nutrients to keep

them alive.

2) The nutrients we need can be divided into five different classes: carbohydrate, protein, fat, fibre and vitamins/minerals. Water is not strictly a nutrient but is nevertheless an essential part of a balanced diet.

3) Each class of nutrient has a different effect in the body, which would not function properly if any of them were missing. Therefore all five nutrient groups are essential to good health.

4) The nutrient groups are required in differing amounts according to their role and uses. Requirements also vary according to a person's age, sex and environment.

5) The five classes of nutrient cannot all be found in one food alone, so a variety of foods must be eaten.

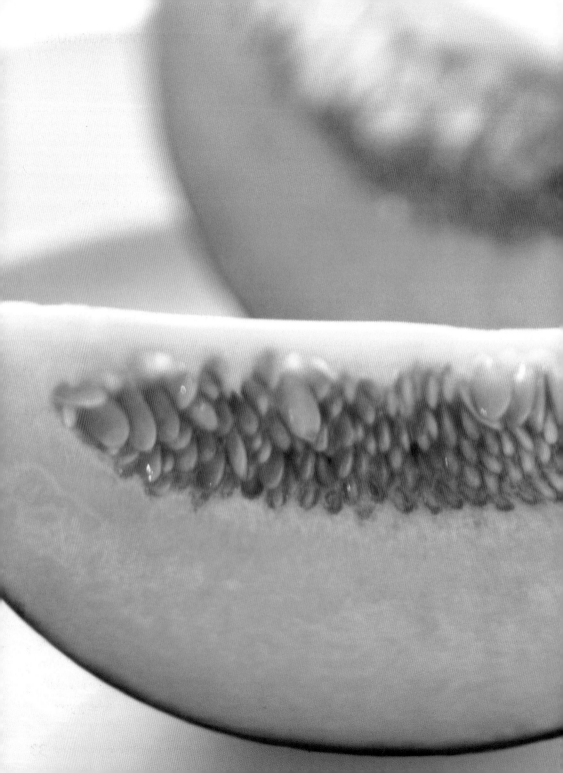

Get Your Balance

While many nutritional principles rely on instinct (such as knowing to drink when you're thirsty or stop eating when you're full) some require a bit more consideration. Eating the right amounts of the crucial nutrients should be as simple as designing a varied diet, but in reality it can be much more complicated – especially when shopping for food also means navigating aisles of processed goods, none of which bear much resemblance to the major food groups. The previous chapter established that the human body requires a variety of nutrients for good health, and this section looks at where they come from and how much of each we should be eating.

As well as a balance of nutrients, our bodies also need a balance of energy. This means matching the amount of energy taken in through food with the amount expelled in physical activity. Whether in the form of relaxing stretches, walking, housework or competitive sport, regular physical exercise is vital to good health. Any programme that offers tips for a healthier lifestyle would be incomplete without recommendations on exercise. In good nutrition terms, maintaining an ideal weight is less about counting calories and more about being aware of the role they play in the diet.

Through processed foods, modern technology has done its best to persuade us that we cannot cook, and that even if we could cook, we wouldn't have the time to. While products such as bread have long been bought from outside suppliers, the range and diversity of processed goods on offer has risen sharply in recent years. It is now perfectly possible to eat three meals a day based entirely on ready meals from the supermarket, although whether or not we would want to is another matter. The final part of this section looks at how to get the most from processed foods, and what role they can play in a balanced diet. Getting your nutritional balance is a skill, like patting your head and rubbing your stomach at the same time, but with a bit of practice it can be mastered for life.

THE FOOD PYRAMID

Anyone who was introduced to the idea of healthy eating at school may remember the food pyramid. This diagram used the point of a triangle to illustrate that the foods towards the top (fat, protein, vitamins and minerals) should be eaten in moderation and those towards the bottom (carbohydrates, fibre) should be eaten in abundance. It may seem simplistic, but this guide is still widely used – particularly in America, where the pyramid has recently been resurrected for a new government healthy eating drive (www. mypyramid.gov).

Although there has been some variation in the pyramid structure over the years – including its radical reinvention as a circle by the UK's Food Standards Agency – the basic idea remains the same: some foods should be consumed more regularly than others. Each new version of the pyramid has been adapted according to current thinking on nutrition, with some emphasising the proportional representation of nutrients and others

suggesting the optimum number of daily or weekly servings. Others still are based on diets from Mediterranean or Asian cultures, which are higher in pulses and legumes and lower in meat. But the one rule on which they all agree is that a good diet should be based on plenty of fresh fruit and vegetables.

The main limitation of the pyramid model is that it encourages the belief that some foods (those given in the highest proportions) are good, and others (the ones given in the lowest proportions) are bad. In both cases, this is potentially misleading. While fats and oils should certainly not be consumed in the same quantity as fruits and vegetables, some varieties have a vital health-promoting role in the body. Omega-3 fats, for example, provide essential fatty acids, while other fats are used in the transport of vitamins. Equally, even though they are excellent sources of energy and should be at the centre of most meals, not all carbohydrates are the ideal basis for a diet. Simple carbohydrates are often less nutritious than complex ones – white bread, for instance, is rarely as healthy as brown.

The FSA's most recent version of the

pyramid, the aforementioned circle (www.food.gov.uk), aims to avoid demonising certain foods by emphasising the importance of nutrient diversity rather than reduction. Called the Balance of Good Health, it breaks down the food groups – like a pie chart – according to their ideal prevalence in a balanced diet. The current guidelines use five separate groups, starting with the two groups that should appear most frequently:

1. Fruit and vegetables
2. Bread, other cereals and potatoes
3. Milk and dairy
4. Meat, fish and alternatives
5. Foods containing fat and/or sugar

A balanced diet should be high in foods from groups one and two, in roughly equal proportions. It should include smaller amounts of foods from groups three and four, and even less of foods from group five. Balancing the diet means choosing a wide range of foods from the first four groups, and occasionally supplementing these, for flavour and variety, with products from the fifth group. Not every meal needs to adhere to the exact proportions specified in the chart, but maintaining this overall balance should be a daily goal.

The FSA hopes to show with the Good Health chart that it is variety that provides the balance in a balanced diet. A limited diet, even one that takes in products from all of the food groups, is not ideal for health. We not only need to pick foods from each of the four main groups each day, but must also ensure that we eat a range of different items within these groups. This is the best way to guarantee a regular intake of all the nutrients we require. It also means that less healthy foods can be eaten in moderation rather than excluded completely.

FRUIT AND VEGETABLES

The five-a-day campaign has long been trying to persuade the British public to increase their fruit and vegetable intake. Given that the average person still only manages a measly three portions per day, this is one area where most of us could probably do better. According to the Balance of Good Health, fruit and vegetables should make up roughly a third of our food intake. This can include dried fruit snacks and fruit juices, as well as canned or frozen products and beans or pulses. Beans, pulses and fruit juice can only count as one portion.

Examples of a portion of fruit or vegetables include:

- Two small fruits such as satsumas
- One medium fruit such as an apple
- A tablespoon of dried fruit such as raisins
- Three heaped tablespoons of peas or beans
- Two spears of broccoli
- Seven cherry tomatoes

Starchy vegetables such as potatoes do not count because they are classified as carbohydrates. Interestingly, while the government's five-a-day guidelines advise caution when choosing canned or snack products with added salt, fat and sugar, the criteria used by the supermarkets for their own five-a-day labels often allow these processed products. According to the supermarkets' claims, baked beans in sugary tomato sauce would count as a portion. The good nutrition recommendation is to check the label, and avoid allowing these products to regularly take the place of fresh fruit and vegetables. For more examples and advice see www.5aday.nhs.uk.

BREAD, OTHER CEREALS AND POTATOES

These should also make up around a third of our daily food intake, although quantities and portion sizes will differ according to age, sex and activity levels. The "other cereals" group includes breakfast cereals, and foods that can be used as the foundation of a main meal, such as rice, pasta and noodles. Oats, beans and pulses also count towards this group, as do plantains, yams and sweet potatoes. Wholegrain varieties, and those labelled as wholemeal or "high fibre", are a preferred option.

MILK AND DAIRY

Dairy products include milk, yoghurt, fromage frais and cheese. They should be consumed in moderation. High fat dairy foods such as cream and butter do not fall into this category. Where possible choose semi-skimmed or skimmed milk rather than whole, and pick lower fat cheeses and yoghurts by checking the nutrition labels.

MEAT, FISH AND ALTERNATIVES

Red meats, poultry, sausages, burgers and other meat products fall into this category. Fish fingers and fish cakes can be counted as a portion, as can tuna and other tinned products. The FSA recommends that we eat two portions of fish a week, one of which should be oily fish such as sardines,

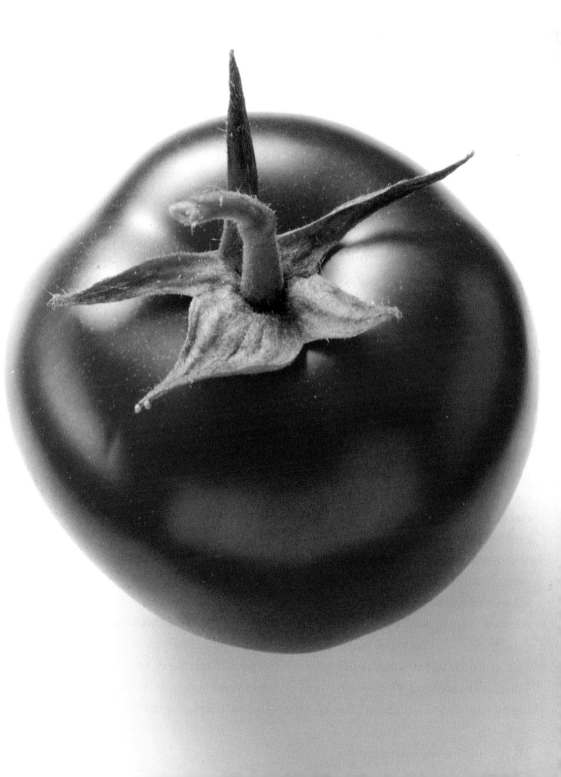

mackerel or salmon. Alternatives to meat and fish are eggs, beans and pulses. While beans and pulses are naturally low in fat, the levels in meat can be reduced by cutting off any visible fat or skin and using cooking methods that do not require extra oil.

Foods Containing Fat and/or Sugar

Fat-rich foods such as margarine, butter, oils, mayonnaise, cream and oily dressings should make up the smallest proportion of the diet. The same is true for sugary foods like cakes, pastries, puddings, ice cream, soft drinks, jams and table sugar. These must form only a limited part of the daily intake, and low fat versions should be chosen where available.

The Balance of Good Health guidelines are an excellent starting point for a well-rounded diet. Put alongside the nutrition information that was given in the Know Your Nutrients section, they can be summarised in the following points for balancing your nutrient intake:

- Variety is key. Eating a wide range of foods from the four major groups given above will provide the best possible range of nutrients. Try new foods or new combinations – it's all about choice.
- Eat in proportion. Try to eat lots of fruits, vegetables and wholegrains, some dairy, some animal or alternative, and a little fat and sugar.
- Fill up on fruit and veg. Aim to eat at least five portions of fruit and vegetables per day – perhaps by including one portion with each meal, plus one snack and a glass of juice.
- Start with starches. Base your main meals around starchy foods, particularly complex carbohydrates such as wholemeal bread, rice, potatoes and pasta.
- Cut the salt. Eat no more than 6g (a teaspoonful) of salt per day. Avoid adding table salt at home, and be aware of the hidden salts in natural and processed foods.
- Avoid dehydration. Drink six to eight glasses of fluid a day to prevent the body from becoming dehydrated, with water taking preference over soft drinks. If you drink alcohol, drink in moderation.

Energy In and Energy Out

A balanced diet is not just about balance of nutrients, but balance of energy. The most obvious determiner of a person's weight is the amount of energy they take in from the nutrients in their diet. Maintaining a stable body weight means matching the amount of food eaten (energy in) with the amount of physical activity undertaken (energy out). Physical activity includes day-to-day tasks, exercise and even the energy needed for internal processes such as metabolism.

Healthy body weight is measured using the Body Mass Index (BMI): weight (kg) divided by height (m) squared (w÷h2). So a person who is 1.7m tall and weighs 70kg would have a body mass index of 70 / (1.7 x 1.7) = 24.2. The result is then compared with a standard chart that shows whether it is within the healthy weight range:

- BMI less than 18.5: underweight
- BMI between 18.5 and 25: ideal weight
- BMI between 25 and 30: overweight
- BMI between 30 and 40: obese
- BMI over 40: very obese

There has been some criticism of the BMI scale because it doesn't always provide an accurate measure of body fat. For example, athletes with a high proportion of heavy muscle may be classified as obese even though their fat levels are actually lower than average. However, the BMI is a useful guide to ideal weight for the general population. An online BMI calculator can be found at www.nhsdirect.nhs.uk.

If your BMI is outside the healthy range then it is likely you are taking in too much, or too little, energy. The energy made available from food is measured in calories. One kilocalorie (kcal) is the amount of energy needed to raise the temperature of one kilogram of water by 1oC, and is equal to 4.184 kilojoules (kJ). Figures for both kilocalories and kilojoules usually appear on nutrition labels, but the ones to watch out for are "kcal", which are known simply as calories. Men need about 2,500 calories per day, and women 2,000.

When food is eaten, the digestive system breaks it down into its components so that they can be used in the body. This is called metabolism, and the three main sources of energy in the diet (carbohydrate, fat and protein) are metabolised in different ways to produce energy:

CARBOHYDRATE

Before carbohydrate can be metabolised, it must be broken down into its simplest form, glucose. This is a more lengthy process for complex carbohydrates than for simple carbohydrates, which is why complex carbohydrates release glucose more steadily into the blood. The glucose is then taken to the cells – for example muscle cells – where it is combined with oxygen that has been brought into the body through the lungs. It is the respiration reaction between oxygen and glucose that produces energy. For each molecule of glucose, the reaction looks like this:

Glucose + Oxygen → Carbon Dioxide + Water + Energy

The energy released in this reaction is put to use in the cells, and the carbon dioxide is transported back to the lungs to be released when we exhale.

FAT

Fatty acids are the main source of energy from fat. These compounds are released when dietary fat is digested, and may be metabolised immediately or stored in adipose tissue to be used later. When energy is needed, free fatty acids are released from adipose tissue into the bloodstream, where they take part in a series of chemical reactions to make them suitable for use. If carbohydrate intakes are low, more fatty acids are metabolised

for energy. However, some parts of the body such as the brain specifically need glucose (particularly the glucose from carbohydrate) to function.

PROTEIN

Once in the digestive system, proteins are broken down into amino acids. Some of these are used to create new amino acids in the body, while the rest are separated into a carbon group and a nitrogen group. The carbon group is used to create energy, while the toxic nitrogen group (usually ammonia) is expelled in the urine. Alternatively, the amino acid may be converted into glucose in the liver. The glucose can then be metabolised to produce energy, just as the body does with carbohydrates from food. Metabolising protein for energy in this way is not efficient, and usually only occurs under extreme stress, or during periods of starvation.

Carbohydrates, fats and proteins provide different numbers of calories:

1g of carbohydrate = 3.75kcal

1g of protein = 4kcal

1g of fat = 9kcal

Of the total energy obtained from the diet each day, at least 50 per cent should

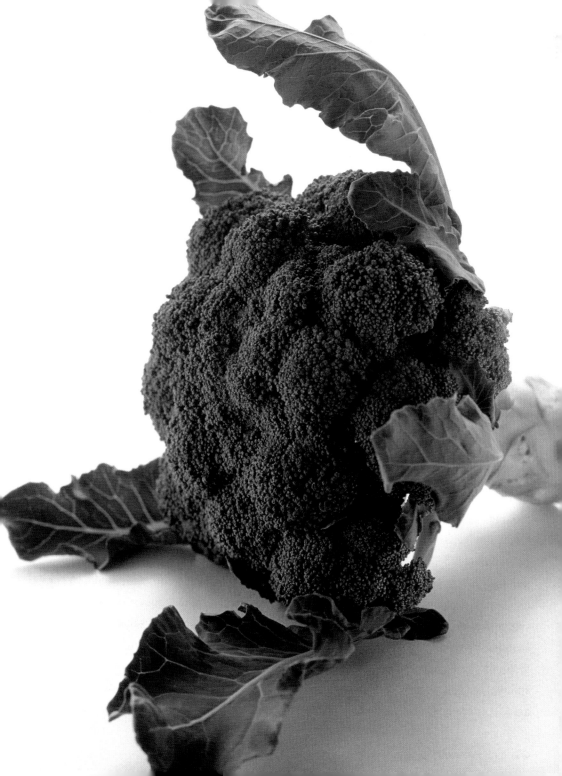

be from carbohydrate, and no more than 30 per cent from fat. About 15 per cent of energy in the British diet comes from protein. Many people don't realise that alcohol is also a high-energy product, providing 7kcal of energy per gram – almost as much as fat.

Equally important to our energy balance is the amount of energy used. 10 per cent of the calories in any meal (its "thermic effect") are taken up in digesting, metabolising and storing the nutrients it contains. All our core processes, such as heartbeat, require energy. The amount needed to keep our basic life functions going is called the resting metabolic rate, and is equal to just over a calorie (4.2kJ) per minute in the average person. On top of this is the energy needed to fuel any type of physical activity, from simple movement to vigorous exercise.

Of the three main energy uses in the body – the thermic effect of food, resting metabolism and physical activity – the latter is the source of the most variation. Physical activity is the area of energy use that we have most control over, particularly in the choices we make over how much exercise to take. Exercise is crucial to good health, and is needed

to maintain strong muscles and bones. There is also a correlation between low activity levels and increased risk of disease, particularly cardiovascular disease and Type 2 diabetes. Exercising regularly can help to reduce this risk.

The Department of Health recommends that all of us achieve at least 30 minutes of moderate physical activity on at least five days a week. It defines moderate physical activity as exercise that results in an increased heart rate, increased body warmth and deeper breathing. The most recent Health Survey for England showed that only 35 per cent of men and 24 per cent of women reached this target.

The 30 minutes of activity do not have to be taken all in one go; three brisk 10-minute walks would count. Activities that encourage strength and flexibility – such as yoga – are also beneficial, and even household chores such as ironing, vacuuming and gardening could be good for your health. Extra exercise doesn't just mean organised sport. It can easily be incorporated into the daily routine, for example by:
- Walking or cycling to work rather than taking the bus
- Using the stairs instead of the lift

- Speaking to a work colleague in person, rather than sending an email
- Leaving the car at home for short journeys

Finding your energy balance involves ensuring that you get the right energy input and output for your ideal weight. For some it may mean increasing their fitness levels. For others it could entail making slight changes to the number of calories consumed in a day. Either way, eating the right amount of food is just as important to a balanced diet as eating the right types of food. Given the rising prevalence of obesity in the UK, it seems that many of us are out of balance.

PROCESSED AND NON-PROCESSED FOODS

Processed goods are the backbone of the modern diet. Supermarkets thrive on them and customers, it seems, can't get enough of them. From bread to biscuits, ready-made lasagne to tinned peas, these products all have one thing in common: beyond a bit of reheating, none of them are cooked at home. While there are plenty of advantages to leaving the cooking to someone else, the disadvantage is that we as consumers forfeit our control over the ingredients. When these ingredients may include high levels of salt, fat and sugar, this is cause for concern.

In general, processed foods are any foods that have been significantly modified before they are put on sale. These might include products that have already been cooked or partially cooked, "combination" foods such as pizzas or ready meals that contain a number of ingredients from the different food groups, and canned or packaged goods such as pies, crisps and yoghurts. Non-processed foods are the raw ingredients of a diet: fresh fruit and vegetables, grains, pulses, nuts and seeds, fresh meats, fish and dairy.

While it would be inaccurate to say that non-processed foods are "good" and processed foods are "bad", there can be no doubt that some highly manufactured foods, if eaten on a regular basis, are not conducive to a healthy diet. One reason for this is their reliance on ingredients that most of us wouldn't even consider using at home. Consumer groups regularly attack processed foods for their high levels of flavourings, preservatives and colourings, often voicing concern about the effects that these synthetic ingredients may have on our bodies. However, by focussing on the issue of food safety they are arguably missing an even more important question: why are these additives there in the first place?

The answer lies in the way these goods are made. Mass production favours cheap ingredients: the cheaper the raw materials, the less flavour they are likely to have, and the more additives are needed to make the finished product palatable. This is one reason why processed foods tend to be so high in flavourings such as salt. Another explanation is that often only small quantities of the key ingredient are used – again for reasons of cost. During a recent healthy eating survey, the consumer magazine Which? found that some chicken curries were under 20 per cent meat, making them almost certainly lower in protein than the home-cooked equivalent.

In cases where the key ingredient is sparse, bulking agents may be used to compensate for the lack of substance and additives for the lack of flavour. Colourings also come in handy to disguise the paucity of ingredients – and to make food that has been through the brutal pumping and refining of the average production line look that bit more appetising. Critics of ready meals describe this artificial recreation of colours and flavours as "food adulteration"; the price we have to pay for cheap, pre-cooked meals.

From a nutritional perspective, the most insidious aspect of this "adulteration" is the addition of "hidden ingredients". These are ingredients that, often unbeknownst to the consumer, appear in large quantities in processed foods. Even though they are listed on the label, the average shopper might not suspect that they are there. The main culprits are not chemical or synthetic additives but two of our most overused flavourings: salt and sugar. Both of these can have serious health consequences if consumed in excess, and are far more widespread in processed food than most shoppers realise.

Bread is a prime example of a product that can contain a significant amount of hidden salt. While a home-made loaf usually requires no more than a pinch of salt, there is not enough time for flavour to accumulate in quick-rising supermarket bread, so salt is typically used as a replacement. Breakfast cereals can also be misleading, with the promise of high fibre and added vitamins sometimes concealing shocking levels of sugar, particularly in products that are aimed at children. It is when choosing these staple processed products that we need to be most aware of what we are eating.

There are currently no official guidelines on how often we should be eating processed foods – partly because there are so many of them, and partly because they play so many different roles in our eating habits. Not all processed foods are additive-laden and free from natural ingredients. Canned or frozen vegetables and tinned fish such as tuna are a simple and healthy addition to the diet, particularly if they contain no added salt or sugar and, in the case of fish, are packaged in spring water rather than oil. While these can be eaten within a varied diet as an alternative to fresh products, other processed foods are best limited, particularly those that are highest in fat, salt and sugar.

In terms of a balanced diet, processed foods should be treated in the same way as freshly prepared meals, with the emphasis being on variety. Choosing products that offer the best reflection of the Balance of Good Health will help to ensure a better range of nutrients. The FSA gives the example of a pizza, which is mostly carbohydrate (the bread base), and also contains moderate amounts of dairy (cheese), vegetables (tomato puree) and meat or fish (topping). Picking a deep pan pizza would mean the meal contains a higher proportion of carbohydrates, while serving it with a side salad would increase its vegetable content.

A bigger challenge is identifying the most nutritious option when the ingredients are not immediately clear – or when the product doesn't automatically appear unhealthy. This is when it becomes important to check the nutrition label, particularly for salt and sugar levels, and also for the total calorie content. A general rule is the more additives, flavourings and colourings a product contains, the more highly processed, and the less nutritious, it is likely to be. The second half of this book gives the information needed to make the best decisions for a whole range of processed products.

One fact to keep in mind when choosing processed over home-cooked is that ingredients make up on average only one third of the cost of a ready meal – the rest is spent on processing and packaging. Needless to say, if the dish were being prepared at home, almost all of the money spent would be on ingredients. We would be better off buying the ingredients ourselves, and flavouring them with herbs and spices rather than chemicals. That way we know exactly what we're eating. In terms of nutritional quality, mass produced goods simply cannot compete with home-made food.

Where it isn't possible to avoid processed goods, stick to the following tips for the best nutritional value:

- Choose processed foods that contain moderate or low levels of fat, sugar and salt according to the Food Standards Agency's guidelines.
- Aim to base most of your meals around fresh produce – even those that include processed goods. For example, if you're having a ready-made lasagne as a main course, serve it with a portion of fresh vegetables.
- Check the portion size. Nutritional information is often given per 100g, so if a portion is 500g you could be eating a lot more of the major nutrients than you expect.
- Check the level of the key ingredient. The most prominent ingredients by weight are listed first, so if the chicken

in your chicken curry appears half way down the list, the product may not be good value for money.

- Look for good quality ingredients – the type you would buy if making the product yourself.

PRINCIPLES OF GOOD NUTRITION

The principles of good nutrition are based on the observation that every nutrient we obtain from food has a role in the body, whether it is positive or potentially negative. Knowing what these roles are and how they can impact on our general health enables us to make the best food choices. Making these choices involves prioritising the nutrients that are most beneficial and seeking to minimise the ones that are only needed in small quantities. It does not mean eliminating certain "unhealthy" groups from the diet or, conversely, picking only the "healthy" options.

If the key to balance is moderation, then moderation is the key to wellbeing. A good diet can help promote wellbeing by providing all the nutrients needed to keep us functioning, but it is most effective when combined with regular exercise and an otherwise healthy lifestyle. The government's advice on physical activity uses this moderation as an incentive, by suggesting that exercise can be incorporated into the daily routine, rather than added onto it. The same is true of a balanced diet: small changes – such as switching soft drinks for fruit juice or reducing table salt at home – can be more effective (and more sustainable) in the long term than major upheavals.

This issue of sustainability is central to healthy eating, which is why pre-prepared foods are included in the recommendations. Processed goods can be used to add occasional variety and appeal to a diet and, if chosen carefully, can be a nutritious alternative to home-cooked foods. The question of which processed foods to buy and how to recognise them will be covered in much more detail in the next section, but from what has been established so far, the rules for a balanced diet can be summarised in the following simple principles:

1) Balance your nutrients by choosing a wide variety of foods from the five major food groups and basing your meals around the ideal proportions shown in the Food Standards Agency's Balance of Good Health.

2) Balance your energy intake and output by taking regular exercise and aiming not to consume more calories than you need per day. For an energy boost, eat slow-releasing carbohydrates, fruits and vegetables, rather than high sugar foods.

3) Balance your intake of processed foods by cooking as many meals from scratch as possible, and eating fresh fruit and vegetables with pre-prepared meals. Pick products that are low in the big three: fat, sugar and salt.

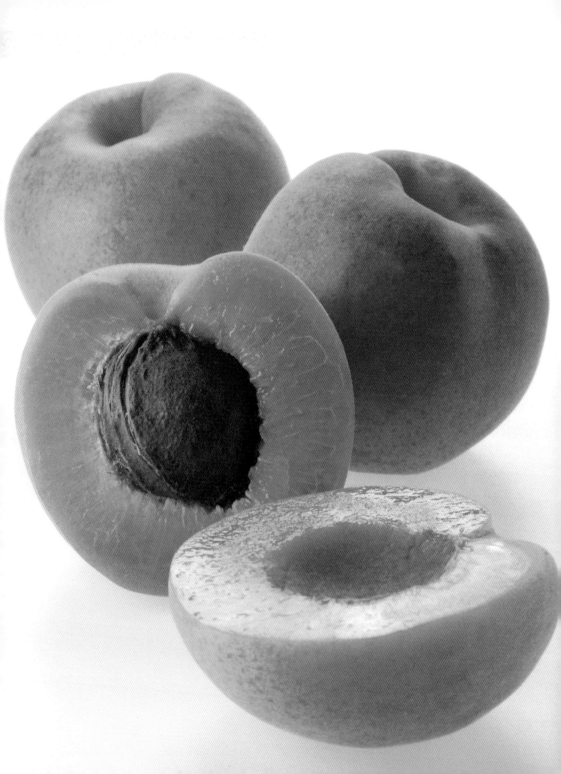

GOOD
NUTRITION IN
PRACTICE

ALWAYS READ THE LABEL •
DON'T BELIEVE THE HYPE •

Introduction

Supermarkets get a pretty bad press. Whether they're clocking up carbon-burning food miles or encouraging shoppers to blow their budgets on TV dinners, the big retailers are often held responsible for much that is wrong with the way we shop for food. While there is more than a grain of truth in many of these complaints, there is also more that we can do as consumers to make the most of supermarkets – and to ensure that they do their bit in return.

Awareness of nutrition is likely to fall somewhere between finding a decent parking space and remembering to buy toilet roll in the average shopper's list of priorities. Although other concerns tend to take precedence, it would be a mistake to suggest that consumers are indifferent to the links between good food and good health: far from it. Nevertheless, the culture of convenience propagated by the major supermarkets has made it virtually impossible to browse before we buy. No one wants to be the person holding up an increasingly irate queue of shoppers while they scrutinise a can of value tomatoes.

As far as most consumers are concerned, supermarkets simply aren't the place for complex dietary decisions.

But this is beginning to change. With the introduction of the Food Standards Agency's colour-coded labels, supermarket customers are being encouraged to take a closer nutritional interest in the foods they buy. The motivation behind these new schemes is twofold: firstly to improve customers' health by drawing their attention towards what they eat, and secondly to provide the supermarkets with an incentive to ensure that their suppliers provide them with healthier products. Label watching – until now a minority sport – is moving into the mainstream.

The eagle-eyed label watcher knows what they're looking for: E numbers disguised by lengthy chemical names; high salt levels given only as sodium; per portion data that vastly underestimates the average appetite. Their prerogative is information, and it's this information that the second section of *The Good Nutrition Guide* reveals. It will put the recommendations from the first section into the context of a weekly supermarket shop, showing how a little bit of knowledge at your fingertips can make checking the label as quick and automatic as throwing your preferred brands in the trolley. There are no lists of additives to memorise, no complex rules for choosing the best products, just practical tips on how to tell the difference between what the labels say and what they mean. And with the help of *The Good Nutrition Guide's* research, all this can be done before you even leave for the shops.

Always Read the Label

FRONT OF PACK

Some of the most important nutritional information to be found on food packaging is no longer hidden away on the back of the packet, but emblazoned on the front. For consumers this can only be a good thing, as it makes checking the label that much easier – it also makes it a little bit more difficult for manufacturers to hide the contents of their products in the small print.

TRAFFIC LIGHT LABELLING

In 2006 the Food Standards Agency set out to design a new labelling scheme that would raise consumer awareness about the nutritional value of popular foods. Its preliminary investigations revealed that the public found standard nutrition labelling confusing, and would prefer that the most important information was signposted in a prominent place on the packaging. From these consultations the FSA developed its "traffic light" labelling system, which enables shoppers to see at a glance how much fat, sugar and salt a product contains. The scheme is voluntary, but by early 2007 it had been adopted by a number of supermarkets including Sainsbury's, the Co-Op, Asda and Waitrose.

Traffic light labels use red, amber and green colour coding to indicate how much of each nutrient is present in a serving of the product, and whether this level is low, medium or high. An amber label would indicate that a food should be eaten in moderation, and a red one that it should be consumed only sparingly. Green-lit products can be eaten more often as part of a balanced diet. Under the traffic light system, a streamlined label gives two main pieces of information:

- The amount in grams of fat, saturates, sugars and salt per serving of the product
- Whether these amounts are high (red), medium (amber) or low (green) according to the FSA's criteria

The criteria behind the colour codes are based upon guidelines drawn up by the EU, and use the following boundaries for foods sold by weight:

	Low (per 100g)	Medium (per 100g)	High (per 100g)
Fat	Less than 3g	Between 3 – 20g	More than 20g
Saturates	Less than 1.5g	Between 1.5 – 5g	More than 5g
Sugars	Less than 5g	Between 5 – 15g	More than 15g
Salt	Less than 0.3g	Between 0.3 – 1.5g	More than 1.5g

For drinks sold by volume, the following boundaries apply:

	Low (per 100g)	Medium (per 100g)	High (per 100g)
Fat	Less than 3g	Between 3 – 20g	More than 20g
Saturates	Less than 1.5g	Between 1.5 – 5g	More than 5g
Sugars	Less than 5g	Between 5 – 15g	More than 15g
Salt	Less than 0.3g	Between 0.3 – 1.5g	More than 1.5g

On the labels this information is given per serving, rather than per 100g, so the buyer can compare the product with adjacent items on the supermarket shelf, and doesn't have to resort to mental arithmetic to work out how much salt or sugar they will be eating.

Additional information under the traffic light system may include the number of calories per serving and how the levels measure up as a percentage of our guideline daily amounts. The FSA's recommendations allow space for supermarkets to develop their own labelling designs, so the presentation of this information will vary from shop to shop.

Despite the support of Sainsbury's and Asda, implementation of the traffic light system has not been free from obstacles. During the discussion stages, supermarkets and manufacturers raised questions over the usefulness of signposting products such as biscuits, which they said consumers already considered "treats", as unhealthy. Perhaps understandably, no business would want to persuade its customers not to buy its products. The FSA responded that the label was designed to appear specifically on foods where the nutritional value may be difficult to gauge, such as sandwiches, ready meals, breakfast cereals and pizzas.

Some supermarkets, notably Tesco, continue to resist the proposed changes, preferring to introduce their own methods of delivering the information to customers. A press statement from the supermarket in February 2006 said: "Earlier customer research by Tesco found that Traffic Light labelling is simplistic and could mislead customers. For example, both cola and apple juice would be colour coded amber for sugar - this is likely to confuse customers who are choosing between these products." Tesco's version of the label includes the same four categories of nutrient but without the colour coding recommended by the FSA. Instead, it gives the totals as a percentage of our guideline daily amounts.

This move has been criticised by consumer magazine Which?, whose research into consumer responses found that the alternative systems used by Tesco and others were "more of a hindrance than a help". Three quarters of the consumers they surveyed believed it would be confusing if supermarkets and manufacturers used different types of labelling, and many found that the inclusion of guideline daily amounts on the Tesco label made it more difficult to understand.

Further criticism came from the National Heart Forum, which accused companies including Tesco, Nestlé and Kellogg's of misrepresenting the nutritional value of their products. One GDA label gave a serving of coca cola as 100ml, even thought the standard can size is 330ml. The NHF also found that manufacturers were using adult GDA figures on products aimed at children, and were adding nutrients such as "wholegrain", for which there is no recommended GDA, to their labels.

As the traffic light system becomes more widespread, the FSA hopes that its red light may not only persuade consumers to reconsider how often they buy certain foods, but may even convince the manufacturers to find ways of reducing the levels of "hidden" salt, fat and sugar in their products. While the scheme may not be flawless, any attempt to bring greater transparency to product labelling should be welcomed. Although it may be a while before we see a traffic light label on a McDonalds beef burger, the scheme

is providing food for thought for shoppers and retailers alike.

BACK OF PACK

NUTRITION PANEL

The standard nutrition panel that can be found on the majority of food labels is actually not obligatory – only if a company decides to promote their product on the basis of its nutritional value do they have to include the full information. Most nevertheless decide to print figures for the "big four": energy, protein, carbohydrate and fat. If a manufacturer wants to put any nutritional details on their packing, these four have to be included.

The other four categories (sugars, saturated fat, fibre and salt) are also voluntary, although they must be provided if a specific reference – such as "low in salt" – is given on the packaging. Manufacturers can also let us know whether the product contains cholesterol, vitamins and minerals, monounsaturated or polyunsaturated fats and starch.

Sometimes the big four categories are placed alongside guideline daily amounts (GDAs). These give an indication of how much of a nutrient should be consumed

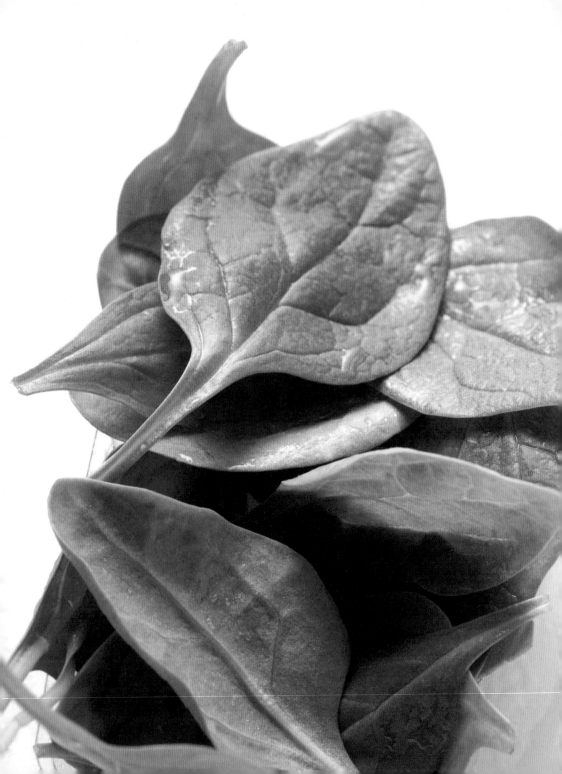

per day. The official GDAs for energy, fat and saturates are given below. There are currently no GDA figures for the other nutrients, but the recommended daily intake figures (taken from Amanda Ursell's book What Are You Really Eating?) give an indication of how much we should be consuming:

	Men	Women
Energy	2,500 kcal	2,000 kcal
Fat	95g	70g
Saturated Fat	30g	20g
Protein	56g	45g
Carbohydrate	313g	250g
Of which sugars	34g	28g
Sodium	2.5g	2.5g
Salt	7.0g	5.0g
Fibre	18g	18g

For the four categories that are of most concern to health, the FSA classifies the following as "a lot" of the nutrient:
Fat: 20g or more per 100g
Saturated fat: 5g or more per 100g
Carbohydrates (of which sugars): 10g or more per 100g
Sodium: 0.5g or more per 100g

The main cause of confusion on the nutrition panel is the difference between "per serving" and "per 100g", with some labels listing the two figures side by side. According to the designated size of a serving, the amount eaten may be much more or much less than 100g.

INGREDIENTS LIST
The ingredients list is given in order of weight, from highest to lowest, at the time the product was prepared. Only in certain cases, such as when an ingredient is pictured on the label, does the manufacturer have to give a percentage amount for a particular ingredient. This means that it is usually impossible to tell exactly how much of each ingredient is present in the finished product. Ingredients lists must include all major constituents, including water, plus any additives, flavourings and colourings that have been used.

There are some exceptions to what the manufacturer has to include in the list: individual ingredients do not have to be listed if they are part of a component that makes up less than 25 per cent of the finished product. For example, if a quiche Lorraine is less than 25 per cent bacon, any extra ingredients in the bacon – such as additives and preservatives – would not have to appear. Similarly, if a product is less than 5 per cent water by weight, this does not have to be stated on the label. Manufacturers are under no obligation to reveal any substances they have used during the production process, including pesticides and medical treatments for farm animals.

However, there are laws to protect customers from deliberate deception and misinformation, which make it illegal for producers to use pictures that are significantly at odds with the ingredients, substitute cheaper ingredients for those given on the label or otherwise mislabel their products.

ALLERGIES ADVICE

One in four people suffer from an allergy at some point in their lives. An allergic reaction occurs when a trigger substance, known as an allergen, is mistakenly identified as a threat by the body's immune system. The immune system responds, causing a range of symptoms such as sneezing and a runny nose. Some reactions are relatively minor, while others can lead to anaphylaxis, a severe

and potentially fatal condition in which the reaction affects the lungs and airways. Although only a small percentage of the population is affected by the most serious allergies, the number of people experiencing sensitivities is increasing year on year.

About a million people in the UK now suffer from food allergies, and many more believe they are intolerant to certain products. Since November 2005, companies have been legally obliged to state whether their goods contain any of the ingredients that are responsible for the most common allergies. According to the Food Standards Agency, the 12 ingredients that have to be listed are: celery, cereals containing gluten (wheat, barley, rye and oats), crustaceans, eggs, fish, milk, mustard, nuts (such as almonds, cashews, hazelnuts, brazils), peanuts, sesame seeds, soybeans, sulphur dioxide and sulphites at levels above 10mg per litre/kilo.

The label might also distinguish between whether a product "contains" an ingredient (meaning it is there in abundance), "may contain" it (meaning that the ingredient is not usually found in the product, but the manufacturer cannot guarantee it is not present) or contains a "trace" of the substance (meaning a very small quantity may be present). It can also indicate if there is a risk of line contamination; for example if a product was packaged in a factory that also processes an allergen such as peanuts. Ingredients that have been so highly processed that they no longer pose a danger do not need to be labelled as allergens.

Use By and Best Before Dates

All perishable products boast a cluster of dates on their labels. The first of these is the sell-by date, which is used by the retailer to keep track of when their stock needs replacing. The second will be either a "use by" or a "best before" date, and it is these that are of concern to the consumer. Of the two, the use by date is arguably the most important. It gives the last date on which the product – if kept in the recommended conditions – is suitable for consumption.

This label is most common on products containing fish, meat and dairy, or other ingredients that need to be refrigerated. Even if a product has not obviously deteriorated after the use by date, it may still be a health risk, so the advice is not to use any product that is out of date. The only exception is if the product is frozen

at home on the day it was purchased, in which case its use by date will be extended by the amount of time stated on the label.

The best before date is not a safety label, but an indication of how long the food will keep before it starts to deteriorate. Most foods consumed after this date should not be harmful, but their quality may be diminished. Eggs should not be eaten after their best before date because of the risk of salmonella.

Labelling Terms

The front of a packet of biscuits is an unlikely place for a minor work of literature, but so eager are some manufacturers to promote their products that the contents are often obscured by extravagant prose proclaiming their freshness, naturalness or authenticity. Although many of the wordier descriptions simply need to be taken with a pinch of salt, others are governed by strict regulations – albeit ones about which few members of the public are aware. This section looks at which claims can be trusted, and which require more careful interpretation.

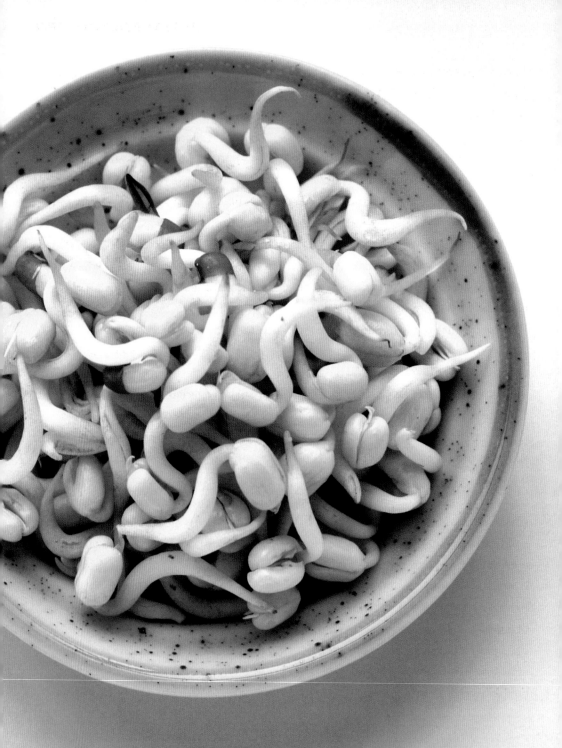

TERMS COVERED BY LEGAL REGULATION
"Low" or "Reduced Calorie"

A "reduced calorie" product must be significantly lower in calories than the standard version. For a product to display the claim "low calorie", it must contain fewer than 40 calories per serving.

"Low Fat" Margarines and Spreads

There are separate definitions for butters, margarines and spreads, which can only be described as "low fat" if they contain less than 40g fat per 100g. A "very low fat" product will contain no more than 30g fat per 100g.

"Flavour" or "Flavoured"

A product that is "flavoured" with something must contain the ingredient in question; for example, chicken flavoured crisps would have to contain real chicken. Chicken "flavour" crisps, on the other hand, need not have been anywhere near poultry – the flavour in question will be entirely synthetic.

"Organic"

For a product to claim to be "organic", it must have been produced according to the EU's legally defined organic standards. These foods will be certified by a regulatory body such as the Soil Association, and must display evidence of this on the packaging.

TERMS COVERED BY VOLUNTARY REGULATION
"Light" and "Lite"

There is no legal definition of "light" or "lite", so their usage varies from product to product. Manufacturers are advised to use these terms only when there has been a significant reduction – of 25 per cent or more – in the nutrient in question. The only way to tell whether a product is truly "light" is to check the nutritional panel. As the statement refers only to the brand to which the product belongs, there is a chance that the regular version of one product may have fewer calories than the "light" version of another.

Low Fat, Low Sugar, Low Salt

To be described as low in fat, sugar or salt, a product should contain less than the following amount of that nutrient:

Low fat: less than 3g per 100g

Low sugar: less than 5g per 100g

Low sodium: less than 40mg per 100g

"Reduced Fat"

For a product to be labelled as "reduced fat" it should contain 25 per cent less fat than the standard version in that product range. As with "light/lite", there is no guarantee that the original wasn't a particularly high fat product to start with, meaning that the reduced product could still be classified as high in fat overall.

"90 per cent Fat Free"

The food labelling guidelines advise against using potentially misleading claims such as "90 per cent fat free", but they still appear on some products. A product that is 90 per cent fat free is still 10 per cent fat – and may even contain more fat than its "low fat" equivalent. The message is only useful if the product is 97 per cent or more fat free, where it is often replaced with the (unregulated) term "virtually fat free".

"Fresh"

The term "fresh" has a number of different uses. It can be used to differentiate between fresh products and those that have been processed – for example fresh peas and canned peas. It also appears on pasteurised products such as milk. Fresh meats and fish are those that have not been previously frozen or processed.

Phrases such as "freshly baked" and "freshly prepared" are more difficult to define, but they should only refer to foods that have been made on the day they are sold. However, as many in-store bakeries simply brown goods that are already part-baked, the term is open to misuse.

"Pure", "Natural"

"Pure" tends to be used on fruit juices, where it refers to the fact that there are no other ingredients in the product. It should not appear on foods that contain more than one ingredient. "Natural" foods are those that are found in nature and, if refined, have undergone only simple processes such as dehydration or baking.

Home-Made

Any food with "home-made" on the label should be just that – the product of a kitchen, not a factory.

"Traditional" and "Authentic"

A product should only be described as "traditional" if it is made according to a process or method that is historically established. "Authentic" foods should have been made using a recipe that is traditional to a particular region, such as Thai green curry or Italian lasagne.

"Garden", "Country", "Ocean"

The regulators discourage companies from using emotive terms such as "garden fresh" on their labels, as they have no generally accepted meanings and can therefore be misleading. It is almost always better to choose a product on the basis of its ingredients and nutritional value rather than relying on phrases, such as these, that are open to interpretation.

"Value" or "Economy"

These refer only to the price of a product compared to other supermarket lines, and give no indication as to the quality of its ingredients. There are no regulations controlling which products can be labelled as "value". The only way to know if an economy product really is good value is to check the nutrition information.

"Suitable for Vegetarians"

There is currently no legal definition for the phrase "suitable for vegetarians" as it appears on food labelling, although manufacturers would be prosecuted if they used the term misleadingly. Consumers looking for extra reassurance may prefer to choose foods carrying the Vegetarian Society's "Approved" logo, as these are independently vetted and only receive certification if they meet the Society's strict production standards.

ADDITIVES AND E-NUMBERS

Additives are so prevalent in modern food technology that the average consumer eats 6–7kg of them every year. They have long been subject to criticism from parents and organic groups, but some added ingredients perform a perfectly legitimate function in the foods we eat. Without additives, we would have trouble producing everything from dried fruit to chicken nuggets: our diets might arguably be healthier, but in terms of processed foods they would also be much less interesting.

All the additives we consume have been passed safe for consumption by the European Union, and appear only in very small quantities in the finished products. The vast majority can be found on the ingredients label. Since E numbers – the standard form of notation for food additives – have become a byword for highly processed, synthetic products, many manufacturers now list the chemical names of additives rather than their numbers. As a general rule, if you don't recognise an ingredient as something you would use at home, there is a good chance it is an additive. While it would be impractical to expect consumers to learn all the E numbers (there are over 500 in common use), an acquaintance with the most popular ones and their uses cannot be a bad thing.

Contrary to popular belief, not all additives are synthetic. Some, such as calcium carbonate (E170), are simply scientific names for naturally occurring compounds. Additives are chosen for their effectiveness in changing the properties of a particular food, be it extending its lifespan or modifying its colour. Each one fulfils a specific role in one of the main categories: colourings, preservatives, antioxidants, sweeteners, emulsifiers/ stabilisers, flavourings and others.

1. Colourings

First impressions of a food are important, and colourings help to make processed foods look more attractive by restoring or enhancing their existing colours.

Colourings are often used to replace natural colours that have been lost in processing, to introduce consistency to a range of products, or simply for decorative effect. They come from one of three sources: a) naturally occurring colours, such as those from vegetables and plants; b) inorganic colours from metals; c) azo dyes, which used to be obtained from coal tar but are now entirely synthetic.

Colourings are identified by the E numbers 100-180. Up to 98 per cent of the colours used are caramels (E150a-d). Bright red cochineal (E120), a non-vegetarian colour derived from the pulverised bodies of cochineal insects, also falls into this category. Inorganic colours such as silver (E174) and gold (E175) may be found on cake decorations. Examples of azo dyes include tartrazine (E102) and quinoline yellow (E104).

2. Preservatives

Preservatives increase the amount of time it takes for a food to go off, usually by preventing the growth of bacteria or mould. Traditional methods of preserving foods include salting, smoking and pickling, while freezing, canning and drying all use modern technology to the same effect. While preserving foods in salt or vinegar gives them a particular flavour, products can be preserved with additives with little or no impact on the taste. Most long-life foods will have been treated with preservatives.

Preservatives are identified by the E numbers 200-285. Sulphur dioxide (E220) is one of the most abundant preservatives, and is used as a coating on dried fruits. Others include sorbic acid (E200), often found in yoghurts, benzoic acid (E210) and its derivatives, and sodium or potassium nitrates, used in the preservation of meat.

3. ANTIOXIDANTS

Some foods go off as a result of a chemical reaction called oxidation, in which fats and oils in the food combine with oxygen from the air. Antioxidants can help to slow down this process, and are therefore used as a preservative in many fatty foods. They are common in margarines, mayonnaises, vegetable oils and meat products.

Antioxidants are identified by the E numbers 300-321. One of the most abundant antioxidants is ascorbic acid (E300); otherwise known as vitamin C. Vitamin E, another antioxidant, is added to margarines in the form of naturally

occurring tocopherol (E306) or its synthetic variants.

4. SWEETENERS

These are used to add sweetness to foods. Of the two main types, the first are "intense sweeteners", which are much stronger than sugar so are only needed in tiny quantities. The second type, "bulk sweeteners", appear in larger quantities as a direct replacement for sugar. Unlike added sugars, sweeteners do not cause tooth decay, and contain fewer calories than regular sugar.

Sweeteners are identified by the E numbers 420/421 and 953-959. Aspartame (E951) and saccharin (E954) are common examples of intense sweeteners and can be found in many sweets and fizzy drinks, alongside acesulfame K (E950) and xylitol (E967). Bulk sweeteners include sorbitol (E420), which regularly appears in low-sugar jams and preserves, and isomalt (E953).

5. EMULSIFIERS, STABILISERS, THICKENERS, GELLING AGENTS

Manufacturers use emulsifiers to allow oil and water to mix. A popular emulsifier is lecithin (E322), which is found naturally in eggs and is the key to the production of mayonnaise. Stabilisers such as carob gum (E410) prevent these emulsified ingredients from separating and help to maintain a consistent texture in foods such as cakes.

6. FLAVOURINGS

These fall into two different categories: flavourings and flavour enhancers. Flavourings add their own flavour to a food, while flavour enhancers don't have a flavour themselves but bring out the taste of the ingredients. The former do not have their own E numbers, but will be listed as "flavourings" on the ingredients panel. They may be naturally produced or entirely synthetic, but as manufacturers do not have to list them by name it is impossible to tell from the label which type a product contains. Flavour enhancers are most often found in crisps, ready meals and other savoury foods, while flavourings appear in a range of different food categories.

One of the most well-known flavour enhancers is monosodium glutamate (E621), which has been surrounded by controversy for its potential health effects on those who are thought to be intolerant. It is found naturally in foods such as tomatoes, but the version added to processed foods is chemically synthesised. MSG is commonly used in Japanese cookery, where it is considered one of the five basic tastes.

Flavour enhancers are identified by the E numbers 620-635. Additives ending in "glutamate" or "inosinate" are likely to be flavour enhancers. Glutamic acid (E620) is used as a replacement for salt, and calcium/disodium 5'-ribonucleotides appear as a flavour enhancer in many snack foods.

7. OTHERS

These are miscellaneous additives that have a wide variety of roles in food production. They include packaging gases, which are used to stop pre-prepared salads from going off, propellants in aerosol cans and anti-caking agents to prevent powdered goods from clumping. Glazing agents add sheen to foods, while firming agents reproduce the solidity or crispness of ingredients that would otherwise soften during processing. Other additives include raising agents such as sodium bicarbonate, and modified starches, which appear in many sweets and juice drinks.

The miscellaneous additives have a range of E numbers, with the majority being 500 or more. Common ones include carbon dioxide (E290) in fizzy drinks, flavouring agent citric acid (E330) and L-cysteine (E920), a flour improver.

Many of these additives have been associated with intolerance, particularly amongst people who already suffer from allergies and allergic diseases. Sulphites (E220-4 & 226-8) have been linked to asthma attacks, and sulphur dioxide (E220) now appears on the allergen label on food packaging. Benzoates (E210-219) are known to cause similar problems. Monosodium glutamate (E621) has been reported to cause headaches, and azo dyes including tartrazine (E102), quinoline yellow (E104) and carmoisine (E122) can trigger allergic reactions including asthma and skin rashes.

The ongoing debate about the link between food additives and hyperactivity in children has led to a decrease in trust around the use and promotion of additives in children's food. A particular source of contention is the fact that there are no laws protecting children over the age of 12 months, even though the use of additives in foods aimed at babies is strictly controlled. Many additives that are in common use in children's foods here are banned in other countries; in the USA, for example, azo dyes including tartrazine have been banned from foods aimed at children. Until the Food Standards Agency publishes the results of its ongoing research into the matter, it is up to parents to choose whether they want to avoid these additives.

A full list of EU approved additives is available on the FSA's website at www.food.gov.uk.

CONCLUSION

Progressive changes are being made to improve the standard of information provided on the average nutrition label, but the food industry has a long way to go before consumers will be 100 per cent confident that what they are eating matches up to their expectations. Much of the problem is to do with companies' (sadly accurate) assumptions that they can use a glossy picture and some fancy writing to distract us from a multitude of E number sins. Finding out what's in a product requires more than a quick glance at the picture on the front, and with the traffic light labelling system this is becoming much easier. As more customers take the time to check the small print, manufacturers will have to become a little less coy about the real contents of their foods.

The information given in this section can be summarised in the following five tips for making the best nutritional choices in the supermarket:

1) Use the traffic light labelling system to gauge whether a processed food is high in fat, saturates, salt and sugar. Aim to limit the number of items that display the red light for one or more of these nutrients. Guideline daily amounts, which appear as percentages on many labels, can be useful as a rough guide to appropriate daily intakes.

2) If you have time to browse, use the nutrition panel for any supplementary information – such as the number of calories or amount of protein. Be aware of whether you are reading the figures "per 100g" or "per serving". Remember that over 0.5g sodium and 5g saturated fat per 100g are high.

3) Unsure whether a product is good nutritional value for money? Check the ingredients. Ingredients are listed in order of weight, so the ones mentioned on the label (the chicken in a chicken curry or tomatoes in a tomato soup) should be right near the top. If they aren't, buy something else.

4) Know that many of the descriptive terms on packaging are only covered by voluntary regulations – or none at all. Be wary of phrases that have no standard meaning, such as "garden fresh". A "traditional" or "authentic" recipe doesn't necessarily mean a more nutritious product.

5) Look out for E numbers or chemical names in the ingredients list. Heavy use of additives suggests that a food is highly processed, and has been made palatable with colourings, flavourings and sweeteners rather than good quality ingredients. A few preservatives or cooking aids is to be expected; a whole list is not.

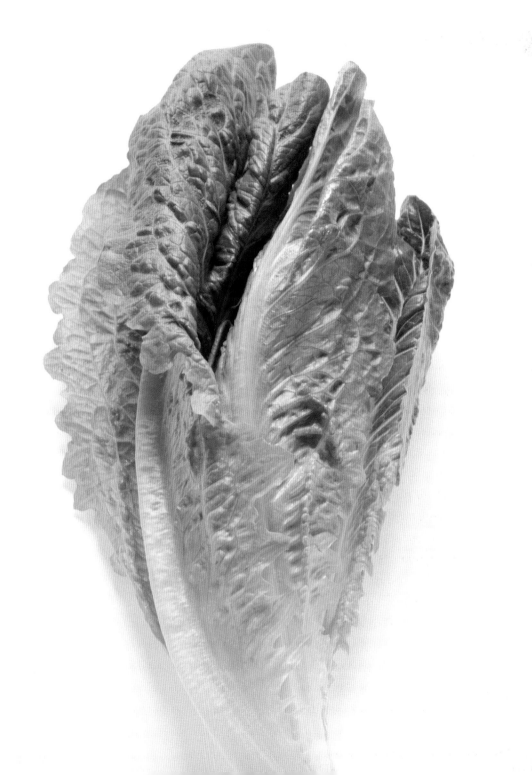

Don't Believe the Hype

INTRODUCTION

Food is a vital part of our way of life. We plan social events around it, celebrate birthdays and festivals with it and use the brief respite of lunch breaks and evening meals to catch up with family members, friends and colleagues. There is so much that is extraneous to the food itself that it is impossible to look at nutrition without considering how it fits into our lives as a whole. This section puts the question of what we eat into context, looking at the outside forces that influence our food choices.

In the last decade, supermarkets have become a major player in British culinary culture. As independent, local shops have died out, the supermarkets have had more and more power in deciding which products are available for us to buy, and in turn in determining what we eat. This would be fine if they sold us only high-quality, healthy foods, but the reality is much more complex. Many of the products they stock are impeccably nutritious, many are not, and with clever advertising blurring the line between the two, telling the difference is rarely easy.

Making informed choices about which processed foods to buy not only involves discovering their nutritional content, but also understanding how mass production – and the structures in place to support it – has an effect on all of the foods we buy. The rise of processed goods can be traced in large part to supermarkets' production methods, and their ever-increasing desire to repackage foods for convenience and novelty. Factory techniques have impacted on every level of the food chain, from animal husbandry to crop selection, raw fruit to frozen vegetables. Our idea of "fresh" food has been permanently altered by the technologies of food preparation, and our expectations of "processed" foods have changed accordingly.

We now look to processed foods to provide more than just a long-life alternative to fresh produce. Canny marketing has helped allow the pursuit of convenience to define our attitudes towards food; for the modern shopper, we are told, cooking is a chore to be avoided and mealtimes are a problem to be fixed. In the marketing materials, and the supermarkets themselves, the culinary solutions to these problems are found. But while we can expect our foods to be processed for convenience, for time-saving, and for functionality, can we expect them to be nutritious?

Before that question is answered in the second half of the book, *The Good Nutrition Guide* looks at how, by approaching it as a business like any other, the savvy shopper can make the supermarket work for them.

SUPERMARKETS

Supermarkets prize customer loyalty above all else, and use many different tactics to persuade us to part with our money at their store rather than the one down the road. From loyalty cards to price reductions, good deals for the shopper always mean better business for the supermarket. In Britain's food economy, the pursuit of profit is at the top of the agenda, and if you believe the critics of supermarket culture, promoting good nutritional values barely figures. Either way, it is true that the big stores' quest for our allegiance has had a dramatic effect

not only on the way we shop for food, but on the foods we buy.

The most striking aspect of supermarket shopping is the apparent level of choice on offer. As food writer Joanna Blythman observes, supermarkets have rendered the culinary world a state of "permanent global summertime", where a vast network of international suppliers has made it possible to buy any produce at any time of year. If you want strawberries in out-of-season November, the chances are there will be plenty of punnets on offer at the nearest superstore. Paradoxically, having such a variety of food at our tables doesn't seem to have improved our diets. Although supermarkets provide us with an abundance of different foods, they also have the power to dictate what these foods are – and in many cases the surfeit of choice is an illusion.

Take ready meals, for instance: the same cluster of companies provides almost all of the products sold in the major supermarkets. The nature of the processes involved in creating cheap mass-produced goods means that there is little room for differentiation. A customer looking for a change of flavour from a different supermarket may be disappointed to find that no matter where they go the meals taste rather alike. When it comes to ready meals, the main difference is more likely to be found in the packaging than the contents.

Indeed, even within individual supermarkets the constant drive for novelty means that the same foods often emerge under different guises. The trick of slightly altering and repackaging products is one the supermarkets use to persuade their customers that the store is at the forefront of gastronomic innovation – and that if they shop elsewhere they would be missing out on something special. So a standard lasagne may morph into an Italian lasagne, tomato soup becomes tomato soup with basil and, on an annual basis, standard meat and dairy products suddenly re-emerge covered in pictures of holly berries and Christmas trees. New products appear before anyone has time to get bored of the old ones, and even if you shop in the same place week after week you will never be in danger of running out of choice.

Traditionally, this sense of ever changing stock was provided by the seasons. If a food couldn't be found in Britain at a certain time of year, it simply wouldn't be on sale. Now that there is "permanent summertime" across the world, most of us no longer appreciate local, seasonal produce. The idea of regional goods has been virtually wiped out by the introduction of food networks that provide a core selection of standard foodstuffs to all the supermarkets all year round. As these networks have grown, supermarkets have encroached further and further into the high street, taking the place of smaller independent retailers and asserting their dominance over our national food culture.

Nevertheless, supermarkets have realised that their customers value the familiar sights and smells of the marketplace, and have begun to introduce miniaturised in-store versions of the town centre. Many superstores now boast their own bakeries, fishmongers and butchers, each proffering a wider variety of goods than even the most successful small business could provide. These atmosphere-defining, "rustic" enterprises are crucial in attracting customers, creating a sense of community that wafts, along with the smell of freshly baked bread, throughout the store.

But is there a nutritional price to

pay for the closure of our independent retailers? In terms of the way we shop for food, yes. The average consumer no longer makes many separate trips to the local shops, picking up a couple of pints of milk one day, some fruit and vegetables the next, and a chicken for the Sunday roast on a Saturday morning. All of the shopping is done in one go, once a week, and it has to last until the next trip seven days later. This demand for longevity has had a huge effect on food production, which, in turn, is having an impact on our diets.

A loaf of bread that would previously have gone stale in two days now comes in "foil fresh" packaging to keep it edible for seven, maybe more. But this robustness is not just about clever packaging; it's about clever ingredients too. Foods as durable as the week-long loaf don't make themselves – they need help from science. Many of the techniques involved in food processing are designed towards precisely this aim: making products that can travel from field to factory to shelf to kitchen with little or no effect on their quality. This may mean using synthetic preservatives or preservative gases to prevent the food from becoming discoloured or going off in transport, or, in the production of

long-life bread, spraying the outside with anti-fungal agents to keep it mould free for longer.

There are legitimate concerns that treating products in this way may have a detrimental effect on their nutrient content. Tests on bagged salads have shown that leaves kept in artificial conditions (known in the industry as modified-atmosphere packaging) contain fewer vital vitamins and antioxidants than those eaten directly after harvesting. Even then, fresh food crops are often harvested prematurely to prevent them ripening before they arrive at their destination, which has a detrimental effect on their flavour, if not their nutritional value.

The intensive growing methods used to cultivate fruit and vegetables involve the use of powerful chemical pesticides, which often end up as residues in the finished products. According to the Soil Association, these fertilisers also increase the proportion of water in fruit and vegetables, producing bigger yields but diluting their nutrient content. Not only this; planting successive crops on the same plot of land can lead to a reduction in soil fertility, meaning lower levels of vitamins and minerals appear in the harvest.

Similar worries surround factory farming. Due to pressures of space and money, animals and birds are nearly always kept indoors and fed on high calorie feeds, rather than being allowed to graze outside. The feeds mean that the animals put on weight quickly, but the meats they produce contain fewer of the nutrients we would expect to find in a grass fed animal. Their living conditions – extremely small, enclosed spaces – make it necessary for the animals to be regularly treated with antibiotics just to prevent them becoming ill. In the case of chickens, a virus in one bird could wipe out an entire flock in weeks. Leaving aside the obvious animal welfare issues, the long-term consequences of eating meat subjected to these conditions are so far unknown, and for many shoppers this uncertainty is argument enough to persuade them to shop organic.

Supermarkets' influence over the foods we buy doesn't just extend to the products they stock, but also the way in which they stock them. The placement of goods within a store can have a dramatic effect on sales, and can direct customers towards certain goods that they might not otherwise consider purchasing. In most supermarkets, fresh produce is to be found at the front of the store, with rows of fruit and vegetables, meats and even flowers greeting the customer as they arrive. Recently, this section has grown to include refrigerated ready meals and other processed foods whose sales benefit from the aura of freshness afforded them by the surrounding raw goods. Behind these are the rest of the processed foods, interspersed with the staple products without which no food shop would be complete. Frequent changes to the in-store layout mean that hunting down these key items often involves traipsing through aisles down which we wouldn't otherwise venture – a perfect opportunity to expose unsuspecting customers to new or unusual product lines.

One of the clearest examples of supermarkets directing their customers' attention towards certain lines is the end-shelf promotion, where buy-one-get-one-free and three-for-the-price-of-two offers are clustered in one place to persuade the consumer to indulge in impulse buys or "stock up" on special offer products. These offers also extend to other retail areas such as CDs, DVDs and books, where supermarkets are able to undercut the higher prices of their rivals, providing them with another chance to show off their cost-cutting credentials.

The stores' biggest discounts work on the assumption that shoppers only remember the prices of a small selection of products. Commodities such as bread and milk, which are purchased on a regular basis, are referred to as "known-value items", and it is from these few that the supermarkets establish themselves as good value for money. What the consumer doesn't know is that a few pence off the price of bread will mean a few pence added to another product; one about which they are less fiscally aware. For those of us whose shopping habits are to a certain extent dictated by these special offers – who can resist a bargain? – this discounting system has a significant effect on what we eat and when we eat it.

There are numerous other ways in which supermarkets make money, one of the murkiest being the "added-value item". This is a product that has been modified in order to offer extra convenience or practicality for the consumer – packaged cauliflower florets, perhaps, or pre-cut carrots. However, the term "added-value" refers more accurately to the returns gained by the supermarket for this redesign of a previously available product: a carrot cut into bite-size pieces can be sold for twice the price of an unpeeled variety. The profit margins on convenience foods are almost always higher than those on fresh ingredients, and it is this that drives supermarkets' promotion of processed goods.

Processing means mass production, and mass production is a guaranteed way of keeping down costs. New lines of added-value items, such as cauliflower cheese or glazed carrots, add variety to the supermarket shelf, and supply the standardised goods that the retailers believe their customers want. As Joanna Blythman notes: "A herd of cattle won't all obligingly provide steaks of uniform dimension." Turn the steaks into meatballs and no one will know the difference.

But just as the use of preservatives can have an effect on vitamin content, so processing can impact on the nutritional value of a product. A survey by Food Magazine in 2005 found that some processed meat products – such as hams and sausages – were up to 30 per cent water. Adding water to foods is perfectly legal, provided it is listed as an

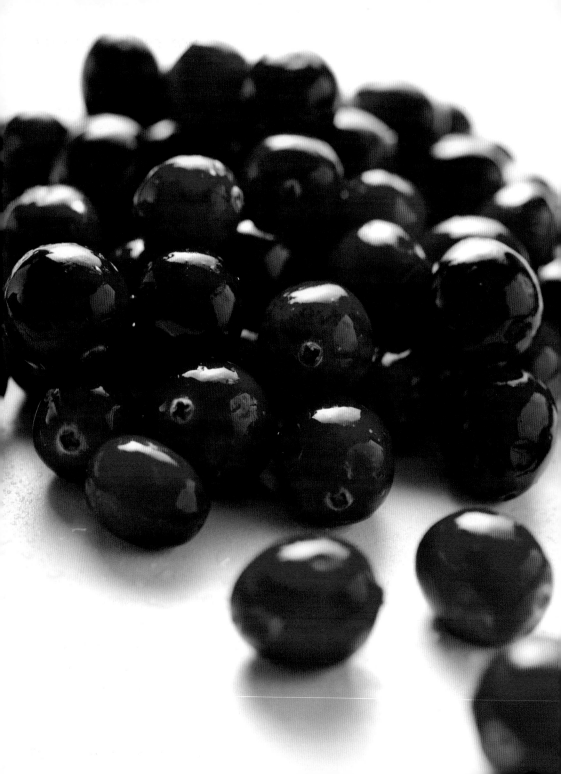

ingredient if it makes up over 5 per cent of the product. Many customers would be surprised to know that they are eating less of the main ingredient than they expected: in an extreme example, Turkey Twizzlers were found to be just 34 per cent meat. Needless to say, the nutritional content of a meat product that contains such a paltry amount of this crucial ingredient is likely to be rather low.

Although the promise of convenience is an attractive selling point, in many cases it would be better, not to mention cheaper, to avoid the "added-value" items and buy the raw ingredients separately. While the nutrition label can reveal a lot about a product and its origins, it cannot disclose all of the processes involved in its movement from the field to your trolley. Recognising some of the tricks of the supermarket trade is a starting point for making more informed choices about the products you buy.

MARKETING

With all these added-value products to shift, supermarkets need to persuade their customers that they are spending their money wisely. This is where marketing comes in. While raw foods are virtually identical wherever you shop, processed foods live or die by their brand. Whether it's an own brand or an external label, the method is the same: associate the food with the desired values, and the customers will keep coming back for more. Advertising permeates all of our purchasing choices, from establishing brand loyalty to encouraging shoppers to try a new product – but only occasionally does it encourage the best nutritional choices.

ADVERTISING TO ADULTS

According to research published by the Future Foundation in 2006, 70 per cent of us believe we don't have time to cook. Can it really be true that the vast majority of the population is too busy even to feed itself? Apparently so: the market for convenience foods and takeaways is booming, and is expected to be worth £12.3bn by 2015. More of us than ever before are eating takeaways and pre-prepared meals as part of our regular diet. Yet the key word in the Foundation's statement is "believe". Whether it is actually true that we are too preoccupied for home cooking doesn't seem to figure.

This common theme, that we have no time to cook and enough money to ensure we don't have to, unites almost all the advertising generated on behalf of processed foods. The "cash-rich time-poor" demographic is the convenience industry's target market, and it has been growing year on year. First it was businesspeople and professionals, then parents, and now everyone from students to part-timers can claim their lives to be too pressured for food preparation. As a marketing technique, it plays upon our guilt that we spend too little time with friends/family/work, and encourages the belief that home cooking is a chore we can happily do without.

One of the ways this translates into sales is through ready meals and other re-heatable, ready-in-minutes "solutions" to the cooking problem. For those who aren't quite ready to give up catering altogether there are "meal suggestions", the helpful back-of-pack ideas recommending that a product is best cooked in conjunction with a number of other items from the same range. A Mexican dish, for example, requires not just meat, vegetables and spices but tortillas, cook-in sauces, jars of salsa and seasonings – all sold separately by the premium brands. Once at home the separate packets combine to give the impression of home cooking, when in fact they are anything but. Meals that should be relatively undemanding to cook from scratch are obfuscated by the promise that the supermarket equivalent is more "traditional" or "authentic" than anything that could possibly be made in the kitchen. Not only are we unwilling to cook, they imply, we are also unable to.

The "cash-rich time-poor" demographic has been further subdivided to create whole new markets for processed foods. Why sell one type of lasagne when you can have a cheaper "value" version, a more expensive "luxury" version, a diet version and a traditional Italian version, each aimed at its own particular market? Even the traditional staples are being redesigned. Something as simple as rice, which once came in bags, now appears in a one-portion microwaveable container: from pouch to plate in one minute for merely three times the cost. Each innovation reinforces the idea that there is a processed food to suit every taste, and that even the slightest of problems can be simplified out of existence. At the supermarket, needs you didn't even know you had can be fulfilled.

The notion of food as a lifestyle choice is essential to the marketing strategies for many processed products, and companies put a lot of effort into establishing a recognisable and associable brand. This may involve all the familiar methods: television and print advertising, internet spots and "viral" videos, special offers and introductory deals. Manufacturers often play up the nutritional value of their product, focusing on one prevalent nutrient, or the fact that the brand contains a fashionable ingredient – pomegranate, perhaps, or omega-3. Some may take a different route, launching their brand (if it is unmistakeably high in fat and sugar) as a luxury item, an indulgence that the busy non-cooking customer has clearly earned in return for their demanding schedule.

Once trust has been established between company and customer, there is an opportunity for the manufacturer to expand into new products – such as the aforementioned microwaveable rice. Successive studies have shown that adults, particularly amongst older age groups, tend to remain faithful to a core selection of brands, particularly those that

they remember from childhood. Given that children can start to display brand loyalty even before they reach school age, companies are willing to spend a lot of money to catch them young. The next section looks at how this is done.

ADVERTISING TO CHILDREN

There are particular concerns about the advertising of high fat, salt and sugar foods to children. Campaigners believe that these processed products can set bad eating habits that last into adulthood. As over a million children are expected to be obese by 2010, it is critical that the issue of junk food marketing is tackled as soon as possible. Consumer magazine Which? has conducted extensive surveys into the ways in which manufacturers target children, and their November 2006 report revealed some worrying trends. While many of the companies claim not to advertise their products directly to under-16s, the researchers' findings suggest that they are in fact using more subtle methods to get their message across.

In a six month period, Which? found 20 different marketing tactics used in the promotion of unhealthy foods to children. Many of these indirect methods

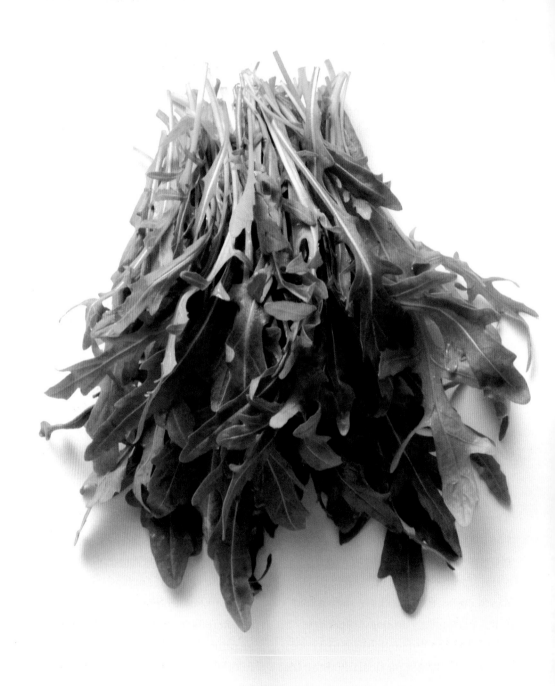

involved processes of brand association, in which foods are marketed as part of tie-ins with new films or television series. These are particularly popular with fast food chains, but also extend to breakfast cereals, crisps, sweets and even baked beans. Others included giving away toys or tokens for collectable gifts with products typically consumed by children. Some companies printed games and puzzles on the back of their packaging, or used national events such as the football World Cup as a platform for launching new or updated products. Celebrity endorsement appeared to be particularly effective in raising product awareness, as was a catchy slogan: the researchers found that children as young as five could recite the tagline for Coco Pops word for word.

Some of the campaigns did avoid marketing to children, and instead advertised to their parents. Most of these promotions made health-based claims for the products – such as "high in calcium", or "contains vitamin C" – which, although substantiated, were often outweighed by high levels of fat, salt and sugar in the product. However, one of the biggest growth areas in marketing terms was new media, particularly text messages and the internet. The majority of the major food and drinks companies now have their own websites, and many of these also run subsidiaries aimed at children. The sites typically include games, stories and downloads – all embedded, naturally, in references to the product they want to sell. Many encourage children to sign up to the site (by giving their email address) in order to access special content and take part in online games and competitions.

Which? felt that some of these campaigns were particularly underhand as they took advantage of media that may be less closely monitored by parents. While even very young children can identify the difference between television programmes and their surrounding adverts, on interactive websites the line between promotion and play is blurred. This concept is particularly alluring to advertisers, as it allows the child to develop a closer relationship with the product – one unmediated by adults. At the moment this type of advertising is poorly regulated, and the codes on non-broadcast advertising have little impact on these viral and multimedia enterprises.

Broadcast advertising, on the other hand, has come under particular scrutiny.

In late 2006, the broadcast regulator Ofcom released a long-awaited report into the television marketing of junk food to children. It recommended that all adverts for "HFSS" (high fat, salt and sugar) products be removed from television programmes aimed at, or of particular appeal to, under-16s by 2008. Ofcom says the measures will decrease the amount of junk food advertising seen by under-16s by 41 per cent, and by 51 per cent amongst under-9s. The move has been condemned by food and drink manufacturers who, along with the TV stations, anticipate a significant loss of revenue as a result of the restrictions.

Nevertheless, there are hopes that the changes may have a positive effect on children's diets, and encourage the companies themselves to cut the number of HFSS products in their ranges. The restrictions may also lessen the peer pressure exerted on children to have particular brands or types of foods in their school lunchboxes, and in turn reduce pester power on parents. If nothing else, by 2008 we will have a better idea of how pervasive an influence television advertising exerts on our food choices.

FUNCTIONAL FOODS

All foods are functional, but some have more functionality than others. Designing foods that have a use above and beyond the one provided to them by nature is a popular preoccupation amongst food technologists, and is often sanctioned by governments keen to enhance the diets of their people. Altering foods to improve their nutritional benefit is nothing new: when rationing posed the threat of deficiency disease during World War II, all flour in Britain was fortified with calcium. Bread flours continue to be fortified today. Similarly, all margarines contain vitamin D by law, and many vegan foods contain vitamin B12, which is usually found only in animal products.

Unlike the functional foods of the 1940s, however, none of the newer additions to the supermarket shelf are introduced under the auspices of a national health scheme. These "functional foods" often appear as the result of scientific breakthroughs or promising research, and tend to be sponsored by the companies that produce them. While a food cannot legally claim to have a medicinal effect (for example in helping to cure or prevent disease), it can be advertised according to its health benefits. The only problem for the consumer is that there is no legal definition of what counts as a health claim.

Some of these claims are backed up with extensive scientific evidence. Plant sterols, for example, have been proven to reduce cholesterol levels by preventing cholesterol from being absorbed from food during digestion. As well as occurring naturally in plants, nuts and seeds, they are now available in margarines and milk drinks as an aid for people who are trying to reduce their cholesterol. These products can be of considerable benefit for people with high cholesterol, but as the British Heart Foundation recommends, they should not take the place of a balanced, healthy diet.

In other cases the evidence is less clear-cut. There has been extensive coverage in the media of research into the effects of omega-3 oils on concentration and learning. Although a number of trials have been carried out on children who suffer from hyperactivity and other learning disorders, more research is needed to substantiate the claim that increased consumption of omega-3 will have an effect on children whose education is not otherwise disrupted. The concentrations of omega-3 found in fortified products such as bread and milk are usually much lower than those used in the trials, and the Advertising Standards Authority has censured at least one advert on this basis.

Another fortified product, the probiotic yoghurt drink, is even more popular but no less controversial. This claims to help reduce bloating and aid digestion by providing concentrated quantities of the essential bacteria needed by the digestive system. Although these bacteria are crucial to digestive health, it has not been conclusively proven that they have a positive effect on those whose intestines are functioning normally – or even that they can survive the journey through the stomach to reach the gut. The only time they are sure to have an effect is if a person is known to be lacking in these bacteria, for example if they have recently suffered from diarrhoea.

While it is best to be cautious when foods promise unrealisable-sounding effects, some long-standing health claims have been fully approved. High fibre and bran cereals are allowed to carry the phrase "helps maintain a healthy heart" for their role in helping to reduce the risk of heart disease as part of a balanced diet. Soya products can help to reduce cholesterol, and are allowed to carry this claim. Some fortified foods, particularly those that contain vitamins and trace minerals, can be a useful supplement to a good diet. Nevertheless, if you are sceptical about a product, save your money and check the evidence for yourself.

ETHICAL SHOPPING

Another area that has been the subject of consumer scepticism is the supermarkets' newfound conversion to ethical shopping. Depending upon your point of view, their pursuit of convenience with a conscience marks either a landmark shift in big business values or a cynical attempt to ingratiate themselves with an increasingly green-thinking public. Either way, the last few years have seen a huge rise in the number of organic, fair trade and local products available from the major retailers. This can only be good for us as shoppers – that is, apart from one problem: the bewildering array of extra choice these new ranges offer. The ethical considerations involved in buying food are extensive and often involve multiple conflicts of interest. Which is better, for example, air-freighted organic produce (with its huge carbon footprint) or non-organic food which has a small carbon footprint but requires intensive use of pesticides? And which is more important, shopping locally to support British farming or buying fair trade products to bring money into impoverished communities abroad?

In most cases there is a reasonable compromise to be found between each of the major concerns, and it is easily possible to incorporate basic ethical ideals into a weekly supermarket shop. To that end, this section will look at what it actually means – in terms of who benefits and where your money goes – to buy fair trade foods, and whether organic produce is really nutritionally superior to conventionally grown crops. In the near future a "balanced diet" may imply not only a nutritional balance, but an ethical one too.

ORGANIC

If going organic is simply a "lifestyle choice" then - as environment secretary David Miliband suggested in a January 2007 interview with The Sunday Times

– it is a choice that growing numbers of us are choosing to make. In 2006, sales of organic produce rose by 30 per cent, with the industry reaching an estimated worth of £1.6 billion. There are many grounds for choosing organic over mass-produced, but with some products incurring a price mark-up of over 50 per cent, it's worth being aware of all the arguments before you decide whether to make the switch.

Miliband's observation that the superiority of organic foods had not yet been proven was seized upon by critics of the movement – and quickly rebuffed by its proponents. For those whose minds have not yet been made up, the organic debate can be divided into three main issues: the nutritional value of organic food, its environmental impact, and its reliability as a genuine alternative to factory farming.

The reduction of pesticide use is central to organic production. An average conventionally grown crop requires regular spraying with insecticides, fungicides and herbicides to keep it blemish-free until it reaches the shops. Campaigners have expressed concern about the "cocktail" effect that residues from these pesticides could have on our bodies. While most of

these chemicals are known to be harmful to humans, what is not known is whether they are harmful in the minimal quantities left behind in our foods – or to what extent they could accumulate in our body tissues over time.

Supporters of pesticide use argue that residues are present in such tiny quantities as to be negligible, and that they are usually found in peels or skins which will generally be discarded before consumption. They also point out that we routinely ingest potential carcinogens – for example, by eating burnt or charred foods – without worrying about any possible risk. There are even suggestions that organically grown produce, complete with its pesticide-free soil, grit and insects, may be more likely to cause food poisoning. Nevertheless, for some campaigners, the fact that the list of pesticides banned for use in the UK is still growing suggests that the safety question remains unanswered.

A similarly contentious issue is the claim that organic food is more nutritious. The Soil Association maintains that produce grown according to organic methods can contain more of the essential nutrients required for good health. It cites studies such as a 2006 report from the

University of Liverpool, which showed that organic milk contained higher levels of omega-3 and other polyunsaturated fatty acids. Naturally, conventional producers dispute these claims – and their reservations have some high profile backers. The chair of the Food Standards Agency, Sir John Krebs, has said that in their view "the current scientific evidence does not show that organic food is any safer or more nutritious than conventionally produced food", although he added that the FSA was "open to new evidence".

This lack of conclusive evidence prevents the key consumer groups – and indeed our environment secretary – from fully endorsing organic produce, but many shoppers nevertheless cite an "instinct" that organic production, by virtue of its "back to nature" approach and refusal to rely on additives, must be better. While it will take more than a combination of instinct and good faith to prove conclusively that organically grown foods are more nutritious, there are plenty of other reasons for supporting smaller farms, of which the environmental and animal welfare arguments are particularly compelling.

Organic farming promises living conditions for its animals that simply cannot be replicated in a factory setting. The lack of space available in factory farms means that procedures such as beak trimming (to prevent chickens from pecking each other) are commonplace, and animals often have little or no access to fresh air. Intensive rearing requires equally intensive use of antibiotics, as an infection in one animal can quickly spread to a whole herd. Organic farms use no growth hormones and resort to antibiotics only when absolutely necessary. The animals are guaranteed access to outdoor pasture and enough space to move about when the weather conditions force them indoors.

These farming methods require significantly more space than conventional techniques, but they ensure that this space is properly managed. Organic farms use crop rotation and pasture resting to prevent soil erosion, and play an important part in wildlife conservation. Buying from local organic businesses lessens the distance from farm to plate, reducing food miles and contributing to the campaign against global warming. But check that the produce is truly local – supermarkets often import their organic food from abroad, even when it is seasonally available in the UK.

More worryingly, there is evidence that the supermarkets are using the demand for organic produce to their advantage, by pushing the boundaries of the label as far as it will go. An investigation for The Sunday Times revealed that chickens were being kept in conditions that fell far below acceptable free-range standards, even though the resultant meat was labelled as "organic" in store. Stories like these do little to promote consumer confidence in organic food – or in the supermarkets that stock it. For now, shoppers need to look for the Soil Association accreditation logo (www.soilassociation.org) or, greener still, purchase fresh foods from local growers. Many farms run weekly fruit and vegetable deliveries, and all will be able to tell you exactly where their produce has come from.

Although the organic debate is unlikely to be settled any time soon, there is one claim on which everyone seems to agree: organic food consistently beats conventional food on flavour. If you are looking for an incentive to eat your greens, there can be none better than this.

FAIR TRADE

When compared to the organic debate, the argument for fairly traded foods seems much more clear-cut. Here, the issues are social rather than nutritional, and centre on the idea that we can support communities in the developing world by guaranteeing them a fair price for their crops. Fair trade products first appeared in the UK in the early 1990s, and since the Fairtrade Mark was launched in 1994 the movement has flourished. The idea of spending a little more for a good cause has captured the public imagination: sales of accredited products increased by a huge 46 per cent in 2006 alone, to make Britain the biggest fair trade buyer in the world.

The Fairtrade Mark signifies that a product meets a strict set of international criteria (see www.fairtrade.net for more information). These ensure that all fair trade goods – whether they come from large-scale tea plantations or small family farms – are bought at a price equalling or exceeding the cost of production. They also guarantee that the producer is paid a "premium" for investment back into the business. Fair trade contracts are long-term, enabling producers to set lasting goals and implement sustainable production methods. Businesses are also assessed for their labour conditions, workers' rights and basic health and safety standards.

Supermarkets have embraced the fair trade ideal almost as readily as consumers. There are now 2,500 individual fair trade products available, including many non-food items such as clothing and sports equipment. Foods covered by fair trade criteria include bananas, cocoa, coffee, dried and fresh fruit, fresh vegetables, honey, juice, nuts, oils, rice, spices, sugar, tea and wine. In early 2007 the major retailers entered into a spirited bout of ethical one-upmanship, launching new fair trade ranges and promising to convert their existing lines to fair trade-only in due course. The "green war" has received a cautious welcome from development campaigners, although certain groups have expressed misgivings not only about the supermarkets' motives, but also about the fair trade scheme itself.

While no one would contend the importance of decent working conditions, the basic principle of fair trade – that growers should be guaranteed a set price regardless of fluctuations in the market – has been the subject of much dispute. Some economists have argued that by isolating its participants from the free market, fair trade makes farmers more reliant on their partners in the developed world. It offers little support for businesses that fall outside the scheme, aiding individual projects and isolated communities rather than promoting countrywide development. Critics of fair trade say that the scheme doesn't go far enough to lift farmers out of poverty, and for some the idea of promoting consumerism – rather than political action – as a form of aid seems inherently distasteful.

Also distasteful was the 2003 revelation that some of the major supermarkets had been exploiting their customers' willingness to pay a premium for fair trade products, by raising prices and taking the bulk of the profit themselves. The Sunday Times reported that fair trade bananas cost on average 74 pence more than the conventional equivalent, of which only 24 pence went to the farmers, and 50 pence to the supermarkets. Recent accusations that the supermarkets are "greenwashing" their reputations, using the halo effect of a few charitable products to overshadow failings in other areas, have dogged the big stores' attempts to improve their ethical credentials. And it's not just ethical groups – environmentalists have weighed in on the debate, pointing out that the resultant increase in air-freighted goods directly contradicts the supermarkets' pledges to reduce their food miles.

Ethical shopping is always going to encounter inconsistencies and contradictions, but as philosopher Peter Singer notes, "it is a mistake to think that because a proposal cannot solve a very big problem it cannot do any good at all." For fair trade, he says, the equation is simple: "If more people buy fair trade coffee, more small farmers can make a decent living from growing coffee." The human rights issues alone should be enough to persuade many consumers to make the switch. A simple rule of thumb for those keen to shop conscientiously is to go fair trade for products that are not grown locally (such as bananas or tea), and go organic for those that are. Whatever your decision, the simple act of thinking about where food comes from, and what environmental and social pressures are involved in its production, is another side to the label-watching discussed earlier in the chapter. In this sense ethical shopping is a fundamental part of good nutrition.

CONCLUSION

Shopping at the supermarket means navigating a sea of distractions. Health claims, marketing slogans and special offers jostle for attention between rows of attractively packaged merchandise and exotic foodstuffs from across the globe. Extracting the most nutritious deals from this tempting selection can be a challenge, but two old adages encapsulate the best of the advice: always take a list and never shop on an empty stomach.

The following is a selection of the most widely used sales and marketing techniques amongst supermarkets and food manufacturers:

1) The supermarkets use numerous means to create an aura of freshness around their products, such as in-store bakeries, butchers' counters and chiller cabinets. Check where your foods have come from: if they have travelled half way around the world, what methods were used to keep them fresh on the journey, and might these have affected the nutritional content?

2) Most processed foods are examples

of "added value", but they don't always represent a good deal for the consumer. Is the new product simply the old one repackaged, or a time-saving gimmick that you could probably do without? Look at the ingredients list to find out whether it actually represents value for money.

3) Before being taken in by the promise of convenience, ask how much time and effort you are really saving by choosing the processed product over the raw ingredients. Is the pre-prepared meal as nutritious as the one you would cook at home?

4) Statements such as "helps maintain a healthy heart" can indicate a healthier choice, but as there is currently little regulation surrounding health claims on food packaging it is often wise to be sceptical. Some links, such as plant sterols and lowered cholesterol, are proven; others are still being researched. Claims should not be misleading, but if it sounds too good to be true, it probably is.

5) There is currently no conclusive proof that organic foods are inherently more nutritious, but "compound" organic products such as bread, biscuits and chocolate usually avoid the synthetic additives associated with their mass-

produced rivals. Supermarkets like to mark up their organic produce, so it can often be cheaper to shop locally. Try farm shops, health food stores and markets for an independent alternative.

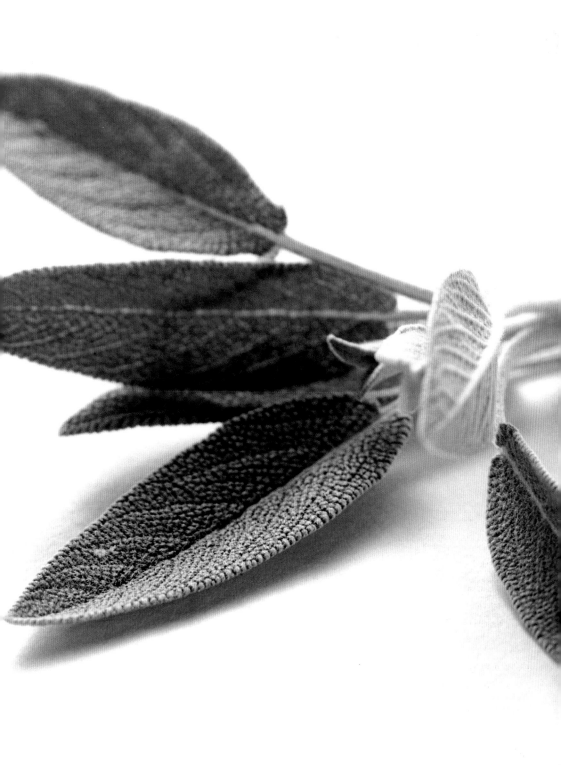

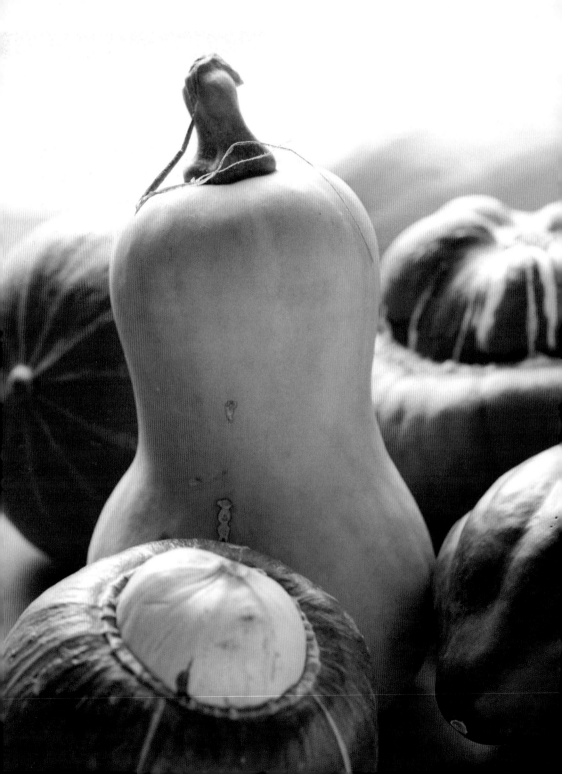

GOOD
NUTRITION
RESEARCH

Using the Research Tables •
Research Chapters •

Introduction

Britain is getting fatter, and our devotion to processed foods is a big part of the problem. We spend three times more on ready meals than any other country in Europe – meaning that a significant number of us are choosing to leave our mealtimes in the hands of big business. And it's not just ready meals; the vast majority of our supermarket purchases, from everyday essentials to occasional luxuries, are mass-produced, additive-filled factory foods. Given the links between bad diet and poor health, this is something we should all be concerned about.

This book addresses those concerns by revealing the truth about some of the country's most popular food brands. The Ethical Company Organisation's researchers have surveyed hundreds of products in supermarkets including Tesco, Sainsbury's and Asda, comparing their nutritional credentials so that you can choose the foods that best reflect your individual dietary needs. While the basic principles of healthy eating are easy to remember, applying them to a shopping list of processed goods and added value items takes far more time and effort – *The Good Nutrition Guide* does all the hard work for you.

First, it rates each product according to whether it receives a red, amber or green light for sugars, fats, saturates and salt under the Food Standards Agency's traffic light criteria. Then it uses these ratings to assign the product a total nutrition score, which indicates both its health value and how it compares to other brands in the same category. Knowing how to "label-watch" using the tables in this book will help you to avoid the products that may be detrimental to your health.

Are "low fat" and "low sugar" items really better than their standard counterparts? How extensive is the problem of "hidden" salt in our food? And is there such a thing as a "healthy" biscuit? *The Good Nutrition Guide* reveals all...

Using the Research Tables

READING THE TABLES

Every chapter in the following section is dedicated to a specific food sector, from baked beans to yoghurt drinks. Each one includes nutritional information about that product category, a table showing the results of the survey, and an interpretation of these results – including *The Good Nutrition Guide's* recommendations. If the product or its manufacturers have been the subject of criticism from consumer groups, or are the focus of current nutritional debate, these arguments will be considered within the chapter.

In all the tables the horizontal axis places the products in alphabetical order according to parent company. This means that all the foods made under a particular brand – such as Nestlé or Heinz – are arranged adjacently across the top of the table. The vertical axis shows the "big eight" figures from the nutrition panel, and gives the product's total nutritional rating. All figures are given per 100g, the reason for which will be further discussed later in the introduction.

At the top of the following page is a sample from the Breakfast Cereals table:

Brand Name	Energy	Protein	Fibre	Carbohydrates	Sugars	Fat	Saturated Fat	Salt	Good Nutrition Guide Score	Company group
Nestle Cinnamon Grahams	411	4.7	4.2	76.1	34.2	9.8	3.7	1.8	25.0	Jordans Cereals Nestle
Nestle Honey Nut Cheerios	374	6.9	5.1	78.2	35.4	3.7	0.9	1.1	50.0	Nestle
Nestle Shreddies	351	6.9	5.1	73.5	15.5	1.9	0.4	0.1	62.5	Nestle
Nestle Shredded Wheat	340	11.6	11.8	67.8	0.9	2.5	0.5	0.0	100.5	Nestle
Sugar Puffs	379	5.3	3.7	85.8	35.0	1.6	0.2	0.2	75.0	Quaker Oats
Quaker Oats	356	11	9	60	1.1	8.0	1.5	0.0	87.5	Quaker Oats

This table shows that even within a single food group there is significant variation in the products' nutritional ratings. It is immediately clear from the figures that some products are less healthy than others, and that many may not be suitable for those looking to reduce their intake of salt, fat and sugar. It is also evident that not all of the foods will be appropriate for diets designed to aid weight loss, help manage high blood pressure or reduce high cholesterol. The table shows that Nestle Cinnamon Grahams, for example, contain higher levels of salt and fat, while Sugar Puffs are low in fats but high in sugar. Most of all, it indicates the importance of making an informed selection: simply switching cereals could increase the nutritional rating of your breakfast from 25 points to the full 100. Such choices

could be crucial in helping you formulate a nutritious, health-promoting diet.

THE CATEGORIES

1) ENERGY

Given in kilocalories (kcal), this is the number of calories contained in 100g of the product. A typical daily calorie intake should be about 2,000kcal for women and 2,500kcal for men.

2) PROTEIN

Gives the amount of protein, in grams (g), contained in 100g of the food.

3) FIBRE

Gives the amount of fibre, in grams (g), contained in 100g of the food.

4) Carbohydrates

Shows the number of grams (g) of carbohydrates, including simple and complex carbohydrates, contained in 100g of the food.

5) Sugars

Gives the number of grams (g) of sugars (simple carbohydrates) found in 100g of the food. This contributes to the total figure for carbohydrates.

6) Fat

The amount of fat, in grams (g), contained in 100g of the food. This figure includes monounsaturated, polyunsaturated and saturated fats.

7) Saturated Fat

The amount of saturated fat, in grams (g), contained in 100g of the food. This figure contributes to the total figure for fat.

8) Salt

This is the number of grams of salt found in 100g of the product. For products that only give a figure for sodium, the amount of salt has been calculated by multiplying the sodium number by 2.5.

The Good Nutrition Guide Score

The last four figures in the table – Sugars, Fat, Saturated Fat and Salt – are used to produce the product's *Good Nutrition Score*. This is calculated from the number of red, amber and green "traffic lights" the item receives according to the Food Standards Agency's definitions. Under this system, a green light for "low" receives 25 points, an amber light for "medium" receives 12.5 points and a red light for "high" receives a mark of zero. The total score is then given out of 100.

For the four categories involved, the boundaries are taken from the Food Standards Agency's Front of Pack Guidance (January 2007), and are as follows:

Sugars (per 100g)

Low: <5 (less than or equal to 5g)
Medium: >5g to <15g (more than 5g and less than or equal to 15g)
High: >15g (more than 15g)

Fat (per 100g)

Low: <3g (less than or equal to 3g)
Medium: >3g to <20g (more than 3g and less than or equal to 20g)
High: >20g (more than 20g)

SATURATED FAT (PER 100G)

Low: <1.5g (less than or equal to 1.5g)

Medium: >1.5g to <5g (more than 1.5g and less than or equal to 5g)

High: >5g (more than 5g)

SALT (PER 100G)

Low: <0.3g (less than or equal to 0.3g)

Medium: >0.3g to <1.5g (more than 0.3g and less than or equal to 1.5g)

High: >1.5g (more than 1.5g)

In the tables, the figures for sugars, fats, saturates and salt are coloured according to the classification they receive: green for low, amber for medium and red for high. Products that achieve an overall score of 100/100 have had their total highlighted in bold.

The total score allows a quick comparison between brands in a particular product category, and indicates which foods are heaviest in potentially unhealthy ingredients. These scores are explained in more depth in the "Our Research Results" section of each chapter. They also form the basis of *The Good Nutrition Guide's* recommendations, which appear at the end of every product section.

GETTING THE MOST FROM THE TABLES

The Good Nutrition Guide tables have been designed to make it as easy as possible for shoppers to compare similar products across a range of nutritional variables. As such it is essential that readers are able to compare like with like, which is why the figures included have been given per 100g of a food, rather than per serving. Individual serving figures (as found on most nutrition panels) are often useful, but they can also be misleading – sometimes deliberately so.

Per serving figures rely on assumptions about the consumer that may not be borne out in practice. For example, many soup manufacturers list a serving of their product as half a can, even though the average soup bowl easily holds a whole can or more. This can lead to distorted consumption figures for "hidden" ingredients such as salt. Presenting the information per 100g gives a clearer indication of a food's credentials, and allows the consumer to adapt the figures to their own diet. To aid in this, each table shows a figure for the "typical serving size" of that food. If your estimated portion size is bigger than 100g, a simple calculation will give the amount per serving: divide the figure for the nutrient by 100, then multiply it by the size of the portion. So if 100g of chips contains 2g of salt, a 140g serving contains (2/100) x 140 = 2.8g of salt.

When using the tables it is worth being aware of some of the techniques employed to reduce the levels of fats and sugars in processed goods – such as replacing high calorie nutrients with sweeteners and other additives. If you are concerned about the quality of the ingredients as well as their calorie content, the figures for carbohydrates, protein and fibre may be of more interest. Indeed, the complexities of modern food production have led to some interesting anomalies, such as certain brands of "diet" soft drink receiving full marks for the four focal nutrients. In these cases the tables are best taken as a whole: while it may be positive that a product contains no sugar, if it also contains no carbohydrates, protein or fibre, it is unlikely to have much to offer nutritionally.

Equally, it is possible for a product that offers good nutritional value to fare less well in the total score. Foods containing nuts or seeds may appear high in fat even though they are rich in healthier mono- and polyunsaturates, while some fatty or salty items – such as margarines and vegetable spreads – have the added benefits of fortification. With this in mind, the "Recommends" sections may be of most value to those who are looking to reduce their intake of added sugars or salt, while others will prefer to take the tables as a whole. Either way, they are an invaluable reference for the conscientious shopper – and a good starting point for label-watchers everywhere.

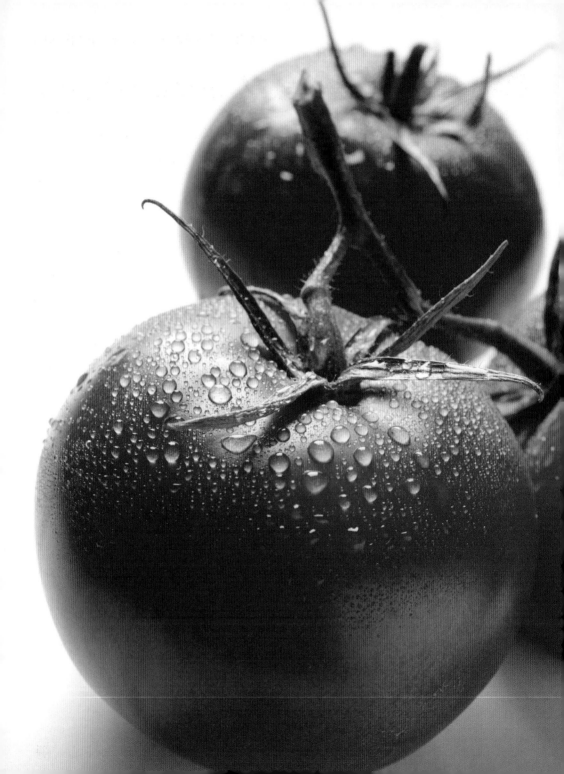

Baked Beans and Canned Pasta

Beans, beans, good for the heart... but not if they're smothered in salty, sugary sauce. Beans on toast has long been a favourite amongst skint students and time-pressed adults, heralded for its nutritional value as well as its simplicity. However, this timeless dish has not escaped the creep of mass production, and some varieties can boast pitifully little tomato in their "tomato" sauce. As a good source of vegetable protein, baked beans are almost always healthier than spaghetti hoops, which in turn have the lead on the much maligned meal-in-a-can.

PART OF YOUR FIVE A DAY?

In 2003 Heinz was criticised for rejecting the government's five a day recommendations on fruit and vegetable consumption in favour of its own strategy: "five a day the Heinz way". The company continued to claim on its website that Heinz processed foods could count as portions of vegetables. According to its criteria, a can of tomato soup makes up two of the suggested five servings, and "just three tablespoonfuls of Heinz Baked Beanz count as one of the five portions of fruit and vegetables we need in our diets each day". Consumer groups have expressed concern that such moves add to public confusion, particularly given that some of the major supermarkets have also launched their own, often contradictory, versions of the five a day logo.

The official NHS guidelines remain generously vague about processed fruits and vegetables, but advise that shoppers should be cautious about which products they choose: "Fruit and vegetables contained in convenience foods like ready meals, pasta sauces, soups and puddings also contribute to your five a day. However, these ready-made foods can be high in salt, sugar and fat, which should only ever be eaten in moderation, so it's important to check the nutrition information on the labels and packaging."

High in Salt, High in Sugar

One reason for the complaints about the Heinz campaign and others is the amount of salt found in many bean and pasta products. While beans themselves are a healthy, high protein food, the sauces in which they are sold are frequently much less nutritious. An investigation for the Food Standards Agency in 2004 showed that one portion (half a can) of some brands of spaghetti in tomato sauce contained over 60 per cent of the recommended daily intake of salt. There was a range of more than 2g between the highest and lowest salt levels in the survey. Considering that the guideline daily intake is only 6g, this is a significant difference.

While there have been considerable improvements in salt levels since this research was carried out, there are still major discrepancies between the different brands. The FSA hopes that today's "low salt" products will become tomorrow's standards, but until then consumers need to be aware that even an established staple such as baked beans can display a huge variation in nutritional value.

This is particularly true of the sugar levels in baked beans and spaghetti hoops.

Some products are surprisingly high in sugar, while others contain flavourings and colours to compensate for the paucity of fresh tomatoes. "Meal-in-a-can" ranges, such as those containing sausages, can also be high in fat and tend to be much sweeter than the average savoury product. Check the small print to see how much meat is found in a tinned sausage.

Marketing to Kids

As a big-selling children's food, canned pastas are subject to major marketing campaigns, most of them aimed at the under-10s. Pasta shapes have evolved from hoops and alphabet letters into the complete casts of popular television series. Not only does Bob The Builder appear on the outside of the can, he can also be found inside – in spaghetti form. TV tie-ins are a crucial source of pester-power for the advertisers, and a source of diversity for the manufacturers.

These products may be invaluable to the parents of vegetable-phobic children, but they are rarely the most nutritious purchase on the shelf. Claims of "added vitamins and minerals" are designed to appeal to those who might otherwise be

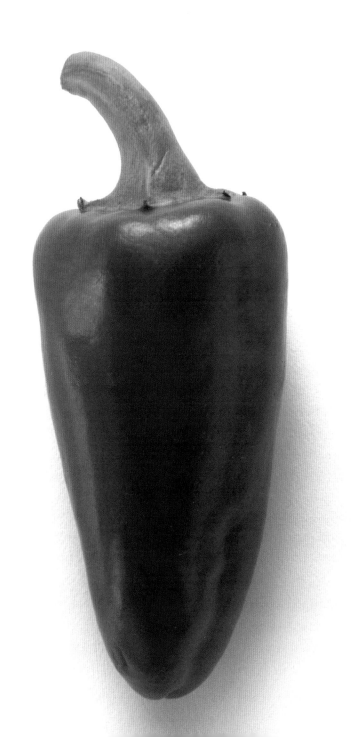

sceptical of heavily branded products, so check the label to see if they have any substance – or whether the benefit is offset by high levels of sugar and salt.

OUR RESEARCH RESULTS

Some brands, particularly La Doria Beans and WeightWatchers Spaghetti in Tomato Sauce, have higher levels of salt, containing over 2g in an average serving of 200g (half a standard can). Although there have been some improvements, salt is still a concern in this product group: a meal comprising a whole standard can of beans with two slices of toast could account for almost a day's recommended sodium intake. Whole Earth Organic Baked Beans come out best with only 0.1g of salt per 100g. Whole Earth is one of the highest rated products overall.

Many of the foods show similar figures for sugars and saturated fats, with the majority receiving a green light for both – but check the packaging to see whether your chosen brand uses added sugars such as glucose syrup. Foods containing sausages or bolognese inevitably have higher levels of fats, saturates and protein. While the cans of beans surveyed contain up to 5g

of protein per 100g, hoops and spaghettis offer significantly less of this nutrient. Pasta products are also notably lower in fibre. Branston Baked Beans are by far the richest in fibre, but also contain a lot of sugars. Their Baked Beans With Sausages contain the highest number of calories.

THE GOOD NUTRITION GUIDE RECOMMENDS

LOWEST IN SUGARS:
WeightWatchers Spaghetti in Tomato Sauce

LOWEST IN SATURATED FATS:
Branston Spaghetti In Tomato Sauce; Cross & Blackwell Scooby Doo Wholewheat Pasta Shapes In Tomato Sauce; Heinz Alphabetti Spaghetti; Heinz Baked Beans; Heinz Hoops; Heinz Mean Beanz Mexican; Heinz Mean Beanz Sweet Chilli; Heinz Organic Baked Beans; Heinz Reduced Sugar & Salt Baked Beans; Heinz Spiderman Pasta Shapes In Tomato Sauce; Heinz Thomas The Tank Engine Pasta Shapes; WeightWatchers Baked Beans; WeightWatchers Spaghetti In Tomato Sauce

LOWEST IN SALT:
Whole Earth Organic Baked Beans

BRAND NAME	ENERGY	PROTEIN	FIBRE	CARBOHYDRATES	SUGARS	FAT	SATURATED FAT	SALT	GOOD NUTRITION GUIDE SCORE	Company group
BRANSTON 50% REDUCED SALT & 50% REDUCED SUGAR BEANS	72	4.6	5.0	12.8	3	0.3	0.1	0.5	87.5	Cross & Blackwell
BRANSTON BAKED BEANS	87	4.8	5.5	16.1	5.9	0.4	0.1	0.9	75	Cross & Blackwell
BRANSTON BAKED BEANS WITH SAUSAGES	100	6.3	4.0	13.4	5.3	5.3	2.3	1	50	Cross & Blackwell
BRANSTON SPAGHETTI IN TOMATO SAUCE	48	1.5	0.7	9.9	2.7	0.3	0	0.2	100	Cross & Blackwell
CROSS & BLACKWELL SCOOBY DOO WHOLEWHEAT PASTA SHAPES IN TOMATO SAUCE	52	1.9	0.7	10.6	3.6	0.2	0	0.2	100	Cross & Blackwell
HEINZ ALPHABETTI SPAGHETTI	54	1.6	1.5	11.2	3.9	0.3	0	0.4	87.5	Heinz
HEINZ BAKED BEANZ	73	4.9	3.8	12.9	5	0.2	0	0.8	87.5	Heinz
HEINZ BAKED BEANZ WITH PORK SAUSAGES	93	5.3	2.7	10.7	4.1	3.3	1.2	1	75	Heinz
HEINZ CURRY BEANZ	96	4.8	4.0	13.6	8.6	1.3	0.1	0.8	75	Heinz
HEINZ HOOPS	52	1.6	1.5	10.8	4	0.2	0	0.4	87.5	Heinz
HEINZ MEAN BEANZ MEXICAN	70	4.5	3.6	12.3	5	0.3	0	0.9	87.5	Heinz
HEINZ MEAN BEANZ SWEET CHILLI	73	4.5	3.6	13	4.9	0.3	0	0.7	87.5	Heinz
HEINZ MEAN BEANZ THAI	93	4.7	3.6	12.7	4.7	2.6	0.2	0.7	87.5	Heinz
HEINZ ORGANIC BAKED BEANZ	72	4.7	3.8	12.8	4.9	0.2	0	0.8	87.5	Heinz
HEINZ RAVIOLI	71	3.0	0.3	12.9	3.6	0.8	0.2	0.8	87.5	Heinz
HEINZ RED LEICESTER MACARONI CHEESE	83	3.5	0.3	11.1	1.6	2.7	0.9	0.7	87.5	Heinz
HEINZ REDUCED SUGAR & SALT BAKED BEANZ	66	4.8	3.8	11.2	3.4	0.2	0	0.5	87.5	Heinz
HEINZ SPAGHETTI BOLOGNESE	79	3.4	0.5	13.2	2.4	1.5	0.2	0.7	87.5	Heinz
HEINZ SPAGHETTI WITH SAUSAGES	88	3.5	0.5	10.8	3.9	3.4	1.3	0.7	75	Heinz
HEINZ SPIDERMAN PASTA SHAPES IN TOMATO SAUCE	54	1.8	0.5	11.2	3.8	0.2	0	0.4	87.5	Heinz
HEINZ THOMAS THE TANK ENGINE PASTA SHAPES	53	1.7	0.5	11	4	0.2	0	0.4	87.5	Heinz
WEIGHTWATCHERS BAKED BEANZ	66	4.7	3.7	11.3	3.4	0.2	0	0.8	87.5	Heinz
WEIGHTWATCHERS BOLOGNESE SHELLS	71	5.2	0.7	9.6	2.3	1.3	0.5	0.7	87.5	Heinz
WEIGHTWATCHERS SPAGHETTI IN TOMATO SAUCE	49	1.8	0.6	9.9	1.2	0.2	0	1.1	87.5	Heinz
WHOLE EARTH ORGANIC BAKED BEANS	81	5.0	3.9	14.4	3.9	0.4	0.1	0.1	100	Kallo Foods
LA DORIA BAKED BEANS	68	5.2	3.7	10.4	5.6	0.6	0.1	1.3	75	LDH (La Doria)

Key

TYPICAL SERVING SIZE: 200G (half a standard can)

All figures are grammes per 100 grammes (expect Energy reading which = Kcal per 100 grammes)

Source: The Ethical Company Organisation / The Good Nutrition Guide 2006 - 2008

For explantion of Good Nutrition Guide Score see the "Using the Research Tables" section

THE GOOD NUTRITION GUIDE BEST CHOICE:

Branston Spaghetti In Tomato Sauce; Cross & Blackwell Scooby Doo Wholewheat Pasta Shapes In Tomato Sauce; Whole Earth Organic Baked Beans

THE GOOD NUTRITION GUIDE WORST CHOICE:

Branston Baked Beans With Sausages

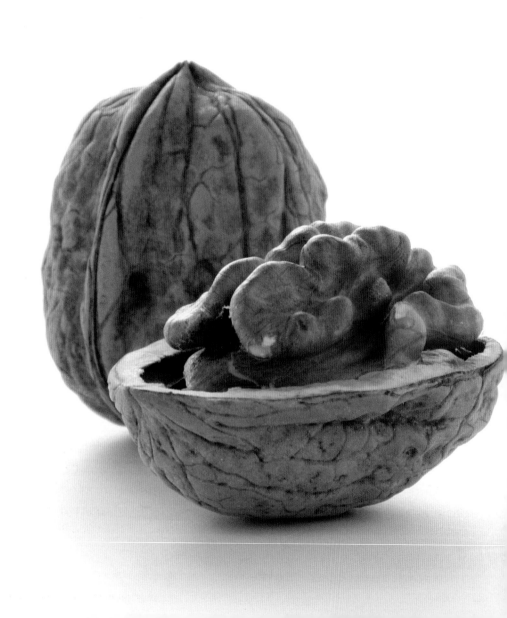

Bedtime Drinks

What better end to the day than a warming mug of hot chocolate topped with frothy cream and a delicate sprinkling of cocoa powder? Bedtime drinks come in two categories, luxury hot chocolates and relaxing malted drinks, and for both types the main ingredients tend to be chocolate, powdered milk and sugar. While all night-time drinks are caffeine free, some brands contain so much sugar that they are more likely to wake the drinker up than lull them to sleep. For the most soporific option, have a look at the table below.

HOT CHOCOLATE AND COCOA

Cocoa is usually made from cocoa powder and water, while hot chocolate is a combination of chocolate, powdered milk and sugar, made with hot milk. The quality of any chocolate drink is dependent on the quality of the chocolate used. This can be determined from the percentage of cocoa solids listed on the label. From a nutritional perspective, those made from dark chocolate are likely to be healthier, as they will contain less of the fat found in milk chocolate.

Dark chocolate itself contains less sugar than milk chocolate, but this doesn't always translate to a low-sugar drink. The manufacturers may simply add sugar or sweeteners to the product to counteract the bitterness of the chocolate. Drinks marketed as "luxury" or "indulgent" are often higher in both fats and sugars than the cheaper alternatives. Higher quality chocolate doesn't necessarily mean fewer additives – check the ingredients list just in case.

PREPARATION

Changing the way a drink is prepared is an easy way to modify its nutritional value. While full cream milk is high in fat, semi-skimmed and skimmed milks are a better option. For an even lower calorie drink, fill the mug with hot water and add milk to taste. If the drink is too rich, simply add less powder.

Some manufacturers give the nutritional value of their drinks per 100g and per serving with milk, but if they don't it can be a struggle to work out exactly how much is consumed per portion. For a rough guideline, a level teaspoon is equal to approximately 3.5g, so an average serving of three teaspoons will be just over 10g – a tenth of the 100g values.

With a little bit more effort, home-made hot chocolate is a good way of knowing what goes into your drink. Choose a good quality dark chocolate and melt a few squares in a saucepan with a mug of skimmed milk, adding cinnamon sticks or mixed spice to taste.

Sugar

Sugar is a key component of any bedtime drink, and in some cases it may even be the most prominent. If sugar comes at the beginning of the ingredients list, then the beverage contains more of this by weight than anything else, including chocolate. Some drinks replace sugar with an artificial alternative, or use additional sugars such as glucose syrup and dextrose to augment the flavour. Unlike artificial sweeteners (aspartame, for example) these are not calorie free, so if you are looking to watch your intake be aware that extra sugars might be hidden amongst the ingredients.

The low sugar content of reduced calorie beverages may appeal, but don't forget to check how much saturated fat the drink contains; if this is high the product may still class as unhealthy. Some low calorie drinks add extra salt to boost their flavour, so even a sweet drink such as hot chocolate could help take you over the recommended daily limit.

Malted Drinks

Malted drinks are made from grains (such as barley) that have been soaked in water, allowed to germinate, and then dried before the germinating plant begins to grow. The processed grains can be used to brew beer and whisky, and also appear as a powder in malted milk and chocolate drinks. Malt is known for its high protein and carbohydrate content, and malted grains are used in many breakfast cereals. However, the amount of protein and carbohydrate in a bedtime drink is more likely to be determined by the amount of milk and sugar it contains.

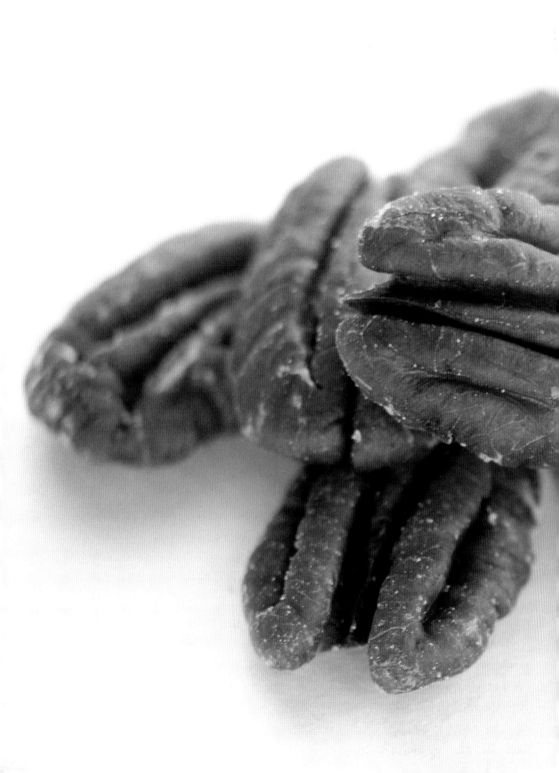

Our Research Results

For sweet products, some of the bedtime drinks surveyed contain an astonishing amount of salt: as much as 4g per 100g in the case of Cadbury Highlights Milk Chocolate. Even though this works out at a relatively small 0.4g salt per serving, it illustrates how pervasive is the use of this hidden ingredient in non-savoury foods. It also shows that choice of product is crucial: Green & Black's Organic Hot Chocolate contains only 0.2g salt per 100g – a mere 0.02g per drink.

There is a similar discrepancy in the amount of saturated fat in these products, with the low sodium Chocolat Charbonnel topping the list at 23.7g of saturates per 100g. In contrast, Clipper's Organic Instant Hot Chocolate has only 1.2g. However, the Clipper product contains more fat overall, with 20g compared to 9.7g for Ovaltine's Belgian Chocolate and Green & Black's 9.3g. As well as having high saturates, Chocolate Charbonnel is also the highest in fat – it is the only product to receive a red light for this nutrient.

The two malted drinks in the table, Ovaltine and Horlicks, both list significantly lower fat levels and less than 2g of saturates. While they have slightly higher carbohydrates overall, these products are about average for sugars. The difference between Cadbury's Hot Chocolate and its Highlights low calorie option is most clearly seen in the sugar figures: Highlights has almost half the sugar of the standard brand. Of the other nutrients, Options Belgian Chocolate is particularly high in fibre, while the two Cadbury products and Clipper's Organic Instant Hot Chocolate contain higher levels of protein.

The Good Nutrition Guide Recommends

Lowest in Sugars:
Caley's ChocLo

Lowest in Saturated Fats:
Ovaltine Original

Lowest in Salt:
Green & Black's Organic Hot Chocolate Drink

The Good Nutrition Guide Best Choice:
Ovaltine Original

BRAND NAME	Energy	Protein	Fibre	Carbohydrates	Sugars	Fat	Saturated Fat	Salt	Good Nutrition Guide Score	Company group
Cadbury Highlights Milk Chocolate	365	17.1	4.6	44.7	28.4	13.0	11.5	4.0	12.5	Cadbury Schweppes
Cadbury Instant Hot Chocolate	425	10.9	2.3	64.2	56.0	14.0	12.4	1.5	25.0	Cadbury Schweppes
Green & Black's Organic Hot Chocolate	374	9.1	9.6	63.5	58.6	9.3	5.5	0.2	37.5	Cadbury Schweppes
Caley's ChocoLo	373	16	8.6	45.9	27.0	13.9	9.1	1.3	25.0	Caley's
Chocolat Charbonnel	528	6.4	9.3	49	49.0	34.0	23.7	0.3	25.0	Charbonnel Et Walker
Organic Instant Hot Chocolate	354	15.5	2.4	68.6	66.6	20.0	1.2	1.0	50.0	Clipper Teas
Horlick's Original	376	10.2	2.8	73.4	40.9	4.6	1.7	1.3	37.5	GlaxoSmithKline
Aero Bubbly Hot Chocolate Drink	414	8.7	5	69.2	59.5	11.2	10.3	1.8	12.5	Nestle
Options Belgian Chocolate	331	11.2	15.5	48.6	45.0	9.7	8.8	3.0	12.5	R Twining & Co.
Ovaltine Original	360	7.3	2.5	78.3	46.3	1.9	1.0	0.6	62.5	R Twining & Co.
Drink Me Vanilla Chai Latte	461	7.4	0	68.7	52.6	17.4	17.0	0.5	25.0	Tea UK

Key

Typical serving size: 10g (three heaped teaspoons)

All figures are grammes per 100 grammes (expect Energy reading which = Kcal per100 grammes)

Source: The Ethical Company Organisation / The Good Nutrition Guide 2006 - 2008

For explantion of Good Nutrition Guide Score see the "Using the Research Tables" section

The Good Nutrition Guide
Worst Choice:

Cadbury Highlights Milk Chocolate; Aero
Bubbly Hot Chocolate Drink; Options
Belgian Chocolate

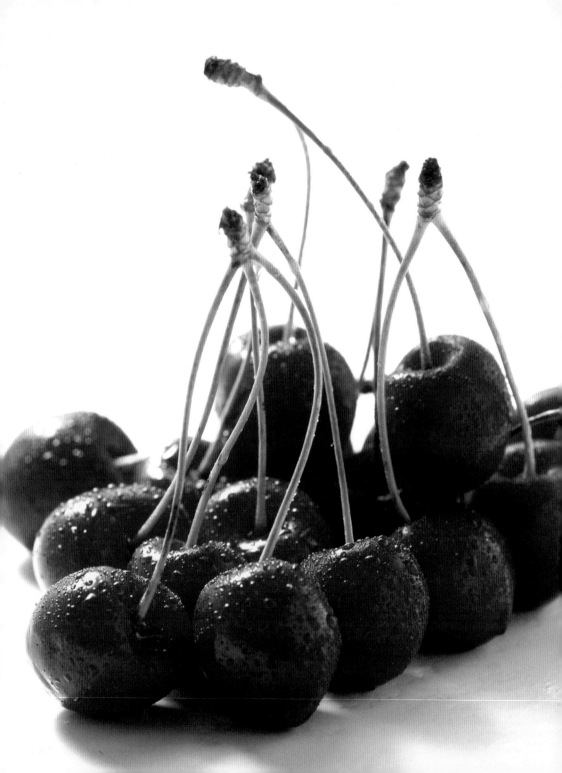

Biscuits

It is a truth universally acknowledged that no tea break would be complete without a garibaldi or three. But is there really such a thing as a healthy biscuit? *The Good Nutrition Guide* compared the credentials of some of the big names in the biscuit world, and discovered a huge level of variation in the amounts of salt, sugar and fat lurking in the average pack. From Jaffa Cakes to crunch creams, this section reveals the best (or, more accurately, least worst) biscuits to dunk in your cuppa.

A HEALTHY OPTION?

Many would argue that the concept of a "healthy" biscuit is fundamentally flawed; after all, a biscuit that isn't a sweet treat is hardly a biscuit at all. Nevertheless, picking a product that is low in salt, refined sugars and saturated fats is often the better option, and sends an important message to the manufacturers about the nutritional value of their goods. Research is currently being done into making biscuits more nutritious by fortifying them with essential vitamins such as B12, but such changes would only be worthwhile if they were accompanied by reductions in other nutrients such as salt.

At the moment, the answer is simply to consume in moderation, or to try one of the less sugary products on the market. These often form part of supermarkets' "diet" ranges, which promise the same taste with lower levels of the most potentially damaging nutrients. However, an investigation by Which? magazine in 2004 found that in some cases the healthy alternative wasn't a positive choice at all. For example, although Sainsbury's Be Good To Yourself chocolate chip cookies contained fewer calories per 100g than the standard version, the biscuits were bigger. Customers who chose the "healthy" option were actually eating more calories than the ones who stuck with the standard version. The best way to make sure you aren't being fooled is to compare the composition values per serving – and to make sure that a serving is equal to one biscuit, not a handful.

(Not) on the Label

Although the manufacturers might like us to believe that each raisin in their cookies has been placed there by hand, the vast majority of supermarket biscuits are made by machine in industrial plants that also produce dozens of other products. For this reason, many brands cannot be guaranteed free from nuts and other allergens. This information should be given on the label. Less likely to appear on the packaging is an acknowledgement that some brands, including McVities, might not be fully GM-free: according to Greenpeace, even if the biscuits do not contain added GM ingredients, any milk (or whey powder) used to produce them may have come from cows fed on GM corn.

Hydrogenated Fats

One other ingredient to watch out for is hydrogenated vegetable fat. This man-made substance (produced by the hydrogenation of liquid oil to give a solid fat) can contain trans fats, which are thought to be an even bigger contributor to high cholesterol than the more widely publicised saturated fats. Having high

cholesterol can increase your risk of heart disease. Trans fats are not yet included in the nutrition panel, so to know if they are in a product you need to check the ingredients list. If "hydrogenated vegetable fat" or "partially hydrogenated oils" are listed, there is a good chance it contains trans fats.

Eating a diet high in insoluble fibre can help to reduce the amount of cholesterol in the blood. Insoluble fibre can be found in products such as oats, which often appear in supermarkets' wheat-free ranges. These may be a healthier alternative, but only if the biscuit is also low in sugar and saturated fat. Beneficial ingredients don't always mean a better overall result: a crunchy HobNob, which is based on oats, also has over 4g of fat per biscuit.

Our Research Results

As expected, there aren't many green lights in the Biscuits table – most of the products receive more than one red light for sugars, fats and saturates, with many receiving red for all three. The figures for salt are slightly better, although Fox's Butter Crinkle Crunch biscuits boast a relatively high 1.3g per 100g. Salt is also

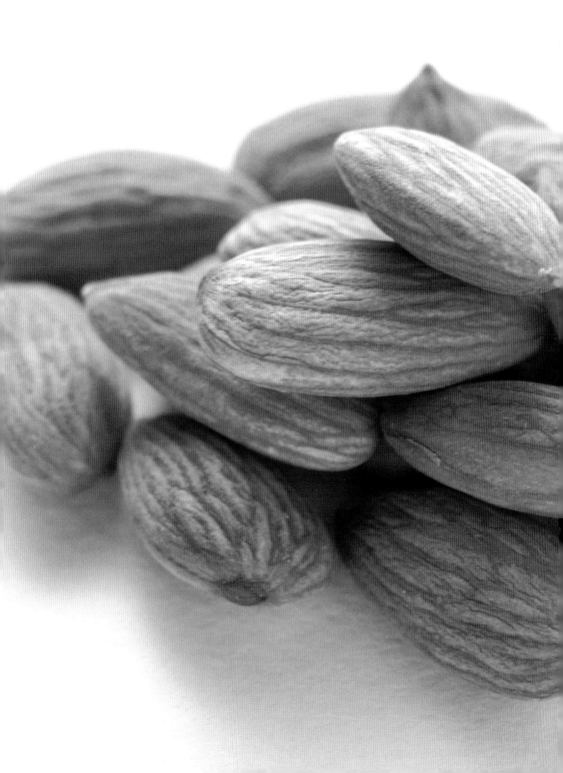

prominent in the McVities range, with their Digestives, HobNobs and Rich Tea biscuits all containing at least 1g of salt per 100g. McVities' low fat option, the Go Ahead Forest Fruit Slice, is also much lower in salt: at 0.5g it contains over half the amount per 100g of an Original Digestive.

Although the Go Ahead product compares favourably to other McVities biscuits, it fares less well against products from other companies. Like for like, the Go Ahead biscuit has similar credentials per 100g as the Jacobs Fig Roll and the Jaffa Cake – neither of which are marketed as diet products. Nevertheless, all three of these, plus WeightWatchers Oat Crunch Biscuits, contain significantly less saturated fat than many of the brands in the table. Top of the list for both fats and saturates is the Cadbury Collection Milk Chocolate, followed by McVitie's Boasters Belgian Chocolate. At the other end of the scale, Orange Jaffa Cakes have the lowest fat content of any biscuit surveyed.

Jaffa Cakes score much less well for sugars, where they are beaten by two unadorned classics of the biscuit market: Original Digestives and Rich Tea. However, neither of these scores

particularly well overall. Amongst the final scores, second place is a tie between Gemme Con Confettura Di Albicocche (Apricot), Jacobs Fig Rolls, McVitie's Go Ahead Forest Fruit Slices and WeightWatchers Oat Crunch Biscuits, while – by a whisker – the Orange Jaffa Cakes come out on top.

THE GOOD NUTRITION GUIDE RECOMMENDS

LOWEST IN SUGARS:
McVitie's Original Digestives

LOWEST IN SATURATED FATS:
WeightWatchers Oat Crunch Biscuits

LOWEST IN SALT:
Baiocchi Hazelnut & Cocoa Filled Biscuits

THE GOOD NUTRITION GUIDE BEST CHOICE:
Jaffa Cakes Orange

BRAND NAME	ENERGY	PROTEIN	FIBRE	CARBOHYDRATES	SUGARS	FAT	SATURATED FAT	SALT	GOOD NUTRITION GUIDE SCORE	Company group
CADBURY COLLECTION MILK CHOCOLATE	515.0	6.4	4.4	56.8	30.1	29.1	18.4	0.8	12.5	Burton's Foods
CADBURY HIGHLIGHTS CHOCOLATE COOKIE CRUNCH	445.0	7.0	3.5	67.7	22.8	16.3	7.4	0.5	25.0	Burton's Foods
CADBURY MILK CHOCOLATE FINGERS	515.0	6.8	1.7	60.8	34.9	27.1	10.8	0.5	12.5	Burton's Foods
ORIGINAL JAMMIE DODGERS	437.0	5.1	1.9	69.5	29.2	15.9	7.5	0.4	25.0	Burton's Foods
FOX'S BUTTER CRINKLE CRUNCH	460.0	5.8	2.4	69.8	31.9	17.5	9.6	1.3	25.0	Fox's Biscuits
MARYLAND CHOC CHIP COOKIES	511.0	6.2	1.3	68.0	34.8	23.9	13.1	0.6	12.5	Maryland
BAIOCCHI HAZELNUT & COCOA FILLED BISCUITS	497.0	7.5	2.5	62.8	25.0	24.0	12.5	0.2	25.0	Mulino Bianco Barilla
GEMME CON CONFETTURA DI ALBICOCCHE (APRICOT)	457.0	6.5	2.0	62.7	32.0	20.0	10.4	0.3	37.5	Mulino Bianco Barilla
TENEREZZE COCOA FILLED BISCUITS	513.0	6.5	2.5	60.9	33.0	27.0	14.3	0.4	12.5	Mulino Bianco Barilla
JACOBS FIG ROLLS	380.0	4.0	3.3	71.4	32.4	8.8	3.9	0.5	37.5	United Biscuits
JAFFA CAKES ORANGE	378.0	4.8	2.1	71.6	51.0	8.1	4.1	0.3	50.0	United Biscuits
MCVITIE'S BOASTERS BELGIAN CHOCOLATE	507.0	5.5	2.8	59.2	32.2	27.7	16.4	1.0	12.5	United Biscuits
MCVITIE'S GO AHEAD FOREST FRUIT SLICES	400.0	5.5	3.7	73.0	33.0	8.8	4.1	0.5	37.5	United Biscuits
MCVITIE'S HOBNOBS	467.0	7.1	5.5	60.8	23.8	21.7	9.5	1.0	12.5	United Biscuits
MCVITIE'S MILK CHOCOLATE DIGESTIVES	487.0	6.7	2.9	62.5	29.3	23.3	12.0	1.3	12.5	United Biscuits
MCVITIE'S MILK CHOCOLATE HOBNOBS	479.0	6.8	4.5	60.7	32.6	23.3	11.3	1.0	12.5	United Biscuits
MCVITIE'S ORIGINAL DIGESTIVES	470.0	7.2	3.6	62.7	16.6	21.5	10.0	1.3	12.5	United Biscuits
MCVITIE'S RICH TEA	453.0	7.1	2.9	71.3	20.1	15.5	7.3	1.0	25.0	United Biscuits
WEIGHTWATCHERS OAT CRUNCH BISCUITS	449.0	7.2	6.1	65.3	22.3	17.7	3.6	0.7	37.5	Walkers Shortbread

Key

TYPICAL SERVING SIZE: 25G (one biscuit)
All figures are grammes per 100 grammes (expect Energy reading which = Kcal per 100 grammes)
Source: The Ethical Company Organisation / The Good Nutrition Guide 2006 - 2008
For explantion of Good Nutrition Guide Score see the "Using the Research Tables" section

THE GOOD NUTRITION GUIDE
WORST CHOICE:

Cadbury Collection Milk Chocolate;
Cadbury Milk Chocolate Fingers;
Maryland Choc Chip Cookies; Tenerezze
Cocoa Filled Biscuits; McVitie's Boasters
Belgian Chocolate; McVitie's HobNobs;
McVitie's Milk Chocolate Digestives;
McVitie's Milk Chocolate HobNobs;
McVitie's Original Digestives

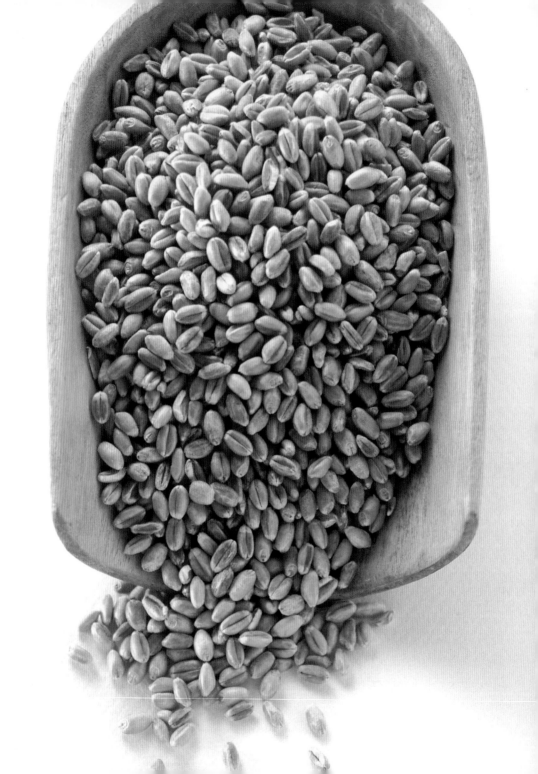

Bread

Supermarket bread seems like good value for money: even the most expensive brands cost just over a pound and in most cases they will keep in the cupboard for at least a week. Unfortunately, the side effect of producing such a long lasting, economical loaf is a dramatic reduction in its nutrient content. The production techniques used for commercial breads have turned one of our healthiest staple foods into a nutritional wasteland. For good value, only wholemeal, organic breads are really worth eating.

THE CHORLEYWOOD BREAD PROCESS

The process that modern commercial bakeries use for making bread has little in common with the conventional techniques of kneading and proving. In the early 1960s a new method of baking was developed, which allowed the dough to be produced in just a few minutes with the aid of high-speed mixers and chemical improving agents. The Chorleywood Bread Process, as it became known, is now used for almost all mass-produced breads.

Although the quick, cheap and easy Chorleywood process has many advantages for the producer, it is not so beneficial for the consumer. Bread used to be considered a nutritional staple, but the majority of supermarket loaves contain hardly any of the protein, fibre, vitamins and minerals that appear in a hand-baked loaf. This is because the CBP allows the use of cheaper varieties of wheat, which invariably contain less protein than more expensive grains. It also allows the addition of large quantities of water to the dough: a Food Standards Committee report in 1986 found that the average loaf of bread was 45 per cent water, and it is unlikely that much has changed since then.

In order for this amount of water to be added, and for the rising process to be reduced to minutes instead of hours, the bread requires chemical intervention from "flour treatment agents". These include improvers, oxidants and emulsifiers that help to regulate the structure of the finished product. One "treatment agent" that may not be listed on the label is hydrogenated (trans) fat. This artificially produced fat has a high melting point, which means that it helps the bread keep its shape even at the high temperatures involved in baking. Hydrogenated fats have been associated with an increased risk of heart disease, but until manufacturers are forced to name all their subsidiary ingredients many of us won't even know we're eating them.

NOT SO "FRESH" BREAD

In an attempt to attract customers through their sense of smell, supermarkets have picked up on an old estate agents' trick: the welcoming and homely aroma of freshly baked bread. Recreating the sensations of a traditional market is a popular pastime for the big supermarkets, and even "local" outlets now have in-store bakeries from which to promote their "freshly baked" ranges. Customers are willing to pay a bit extra for something that has been produced on the same day, and assume that they are getting the service they would expect from an

independent bakers.

Sometimes this may be true, but in most cases "fresh" supermarket bread is not baked but "baked-off"; it arrives in the store as a partially cooked, frozen dough and is then crisped and browned on site, ready for sale. Industry figures suggest that half of in-store bakeries make their breads in this way. Nearly all of the rest will use a pre-prepared bread mix to save on cooking time. In nutritional terms these loaves are unlikely to be much better than the packaged varieties. They will also contain a similar number of treatment agents – only here they will be used to prolong the life of the bread before it is baked, rather than after.

BREAD WARS

In 1999 the supermarkets embarked on a price war that left a loaf of own brand white bread costing as little as a handful of penny sweets. At the height of the competition, Kwik Save, Asda and Tesco reduced their cheapest loaves to just 7p, sparking outcry from union leaders and small retailers. While this was an extreme case, it highlights how important the bread market is to the supermarkets – and why it is crucial that shoppers look beyond the price label.

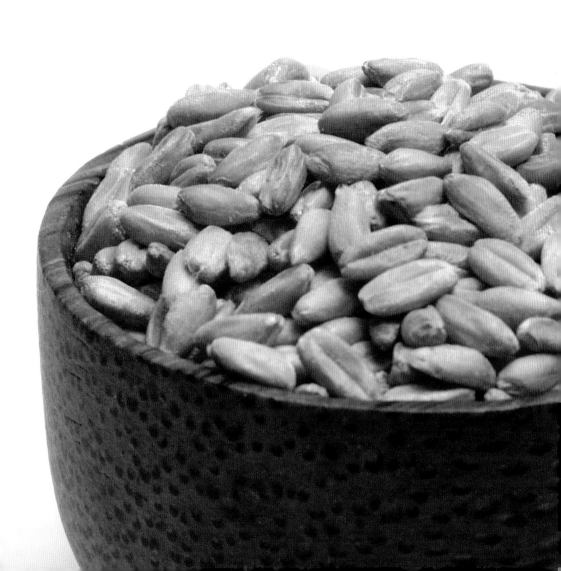

OUR RESEARCH RESULTS

One of the main concerns surrounding shop-bought breads is their high salt content, so it is perhaps surprising that the difference between the most and least salty breads in the table is relatively small. While Burgen Soya & Linseed and Nimble Malted Wholegrain have the least salt at 0.8g per 100g, only 0.5g more gives Kingsmill Head Start With Omega-3 White, Kingsmill Soft White Rolls, Hovis Farmhouse White and Warburtons White Batch the highest figures at 1.3g per 100g. Nevertheless, two rounds of sandwiches (each with two slices of bread) from these saltier loaves would amount to almost half the recommended daily intake of sodium – more if the sandwich included a salty filling such as cheese or Marmite.

Although the majority of the breads surveyed contain very little fat or saturates, a few loaves receive amber lights for these nutrients. In the cases of Allinson Sunflower Multigrain, Burgen Soya & Linseed and Warburtons Seeded Batch, for example, the extra fats are explained by the (nutritionally valuable) mono- and polyunsaturates found in their added seeds – for others more caution

is advised. In most cases, the fibre and protein levels may give the most useful indication of the quality of flour used.

THE GOOD NUTRITION GUIDE RECOMMENDS

LOWEST IN SUGARS:
Kingsmill Soft White Rolls; Hovis Invisible Crust White; Hovis Supreme White

LOWEST IN SATURATED FATS:
Hovis Supreme White

LOWEST IN SALT:
Burgen Soya & Linseed; Nimble Malted Wholegrain

THE GOOD NUTRITION GUIDE BEST CHOICE:
[Many on 87.5]

THE GOOD NUTRITION GUIDE WORST CHOICE:
Burgen Soya & Linseed; Country Miller Organic White Rolls; Warburtons Seeded Batch

BREAD

Brand Name	Energy	Protein	Fibre	Carbohydrates	Sugars	Fat	Saturated Fat	Salt	Good Nutrition Guide Score	Company group
Burgen Soya & Linseed	274	15.9	6.8	29.8	5.4	10.1	1.4	0.8	62.5	Allied Bakeries
Kingsmill Crusts Away White	222	8	2.8	43.3	3.3	1.9	0.3	1.1	87.5	Allied Bakeries
Kingsmill Crusts Away 50 - 50	211	8.8	3.7	38.2	3.5	2.5	0.4	1.0	87.5	Allied Bakeries
Kingsmill 50 - 50 with omega 3	225	9.9	4.9	41.2	3.4	2.3	0.4	1.0	87.5	Allied Bakeries
Kingsmill Soft White Rolls	250	9.3	2.9	44	1.0	4.1	1.5	1.3	75.0	Allied Bakeries
Kingsmill Square White	232	8.8	2.8	43.8	2.7	2.4	0.4	1.2	87.5	Allied Bakeries
Kingsmill love to toast White	234	9.3	3.1	42.3	2.5	3.1	0.6	1.0	75.0	Allied Bakeries
Kingsmill Wholemeal	221	10.1	6.8	37.6	3.3	3.4	0.6	1.0	75.0	Allied Bakeries
Country Miller Organic White Rolls	278	9.2	2.2	51.9	2.6	3.7	1.7	1.0	62.5	Nicholas & Harris Ltd
Hovis Best of Both	220	9.1	4.6	40.9	4.0	2.2	0.5	1.1	87.5	Premier Foods
Hovis Country Granary	218	11.1	6.5	37	1.9	2.9	0.6	1.0	87.5	Premier Foods
Hovis Farmhouse White	226	8.3	3.3	44.7	3.4	1.7	0.3	1.3	87.5	Premier Foods
Hovis Farmhouse Wholemeal	207	11	7.1	36	3.6	2.2	0.4	1.1	87.5	Premier Foods
Hovis Granary	231	9.2	3.8	44.8	2.7	1.7	0.3	1.2	87.5	Premier Foods
Hovis Invisible Crust Best Of Both	223	9.7	4.4	41.3	1.6	2.1	0.5	1.1	87.5	Premier Foods
Hovis Invisible Crust White	226	8.8	2.4	44.1	1.0	1.6	0.3	1.2	87.5	Premier Foods
Hovis Oatmeal Granary	236	9.2	3.1	45.3	2.7	2.1	0.4	1.2	87.5	Premier Foods
Hovis Original Wheatgerm	214	10	5.3	38.6	3.1	2.2	0.4	1.0	87.5	Premier Foods
Hovis Square White	231	8.5	2.6	44.7	4.1	2.0	0.5	1.2	87.5	Premier Foods
Hovis Sunflower Granary	271	10.1	2.9	44.9	2.2	5.7	0.7	1.1	75.0	Premier Foods
Hovis Supreme White	222	9.2	2.9	42.9	1.0	1.5	0.2	1.2	87.5	Premier Foods
Hovis White Granary	248	10.9	3.8	41.7	1.4	4.2	0.5	1.2	87.5	Premier Foods
Hovis Wholemeal	227	11.4	6.5	40.3	3.7	2.3	0.5	1.0	87.5	Premier Foods
Nimble Malted Wholegrain	222	10.4	6.7	41.9	2.7	1.4	0.3	0.8	87.5	Premier Foods
Nimble White	219	10.1	7.5	40.6	2.7	1.8	0.4	0.9	87.5	Premier Foods
Nimble Wholemeal	219	12.2	6.8	37	2.2	2.5	0.5	1.1	87.5	Premier Foods
Warburtons Farmhouse Soft White	236	9.9	2.7	43.4	1.7	2.5	1.0	1.2	87.5	Warburtons
Warburtons Medium White	234	9.9	2.6	43.8	2.2	2.0	0.7	1.2	87.5	Warburtons
Warburtons Sandwich Rolls	258	9.7	2.4	44.6	2.3	4.5	1.2	1.2	75.0	Warburtons
Warburtons Seeded Batch	288	12.3	6	39.7	3.2	8.9	1.9	1.2	62.5	Warburtons
Warburtons Stoneground Wholemeal	210	10.3	6.9	35.7	2.3	2.6	0.9	1.2	87.5	Warburtons
Warburtons White Batch	223	8.7	2.5	43.1	1.8	1.9	0.9	1.3	87.5	Warburtons
Warburtons Wholegrain Goodness	232	10.9	6.3	38.4	2.9	3.9	0.8	1.0	75.0	Warburtons
WeightWatchers Brown Danish	215	11	7.3	38.4	2.1	1.8	0.7	1.2	87.5	Warburtons
WeightWatchers Malted Danish	241	12.4	4.2	44.5	2.6	1.6	0.6	1.2	87.5	Warburtons

Key

TYPICAL SERVING SIZE: **100g**

All figures are grammes per 100 grammes (expect Energy reading which = Kcal per100 grammes)

Source: The Ethical Company Organisation / The Good Nutrition Guide 2006 - 2008

For explantion of Good Nutrition Guide Score see the "Using the Research Tables" section

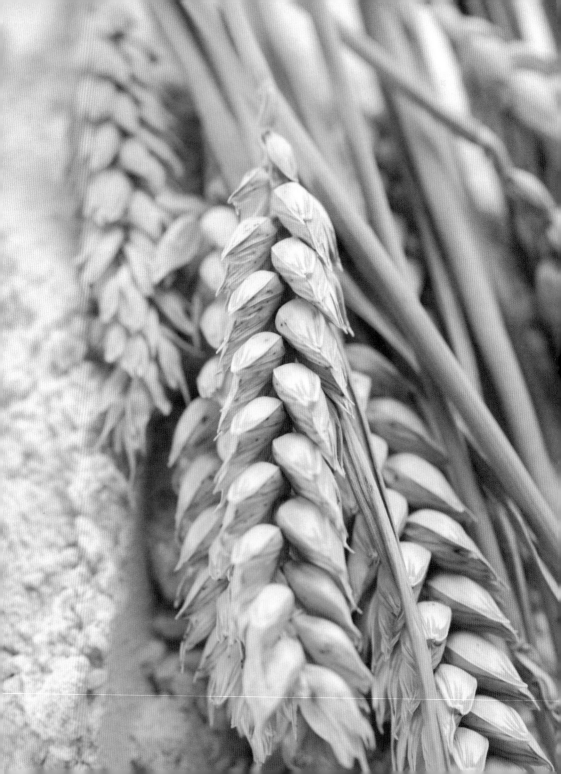

Breakfast Cereals

Given the choice between a bacon butty and a bowl of cereal, most of us would pick the cereal as the healthier option. But most of us, it seems, might be wrong. Some cereals contain as much sugar as a chocolate bar and as much saturated fat as a cake – something no quantity of added vitamins and minerals is going to rectify. Breakfast is the only time of day when a single item can count for an entire meal, so a nutritious cereal is imperative to a healthy diet. The following chapter singles out the best.

WHAT GOES INTO YOUR CEREAL?

Most breakfast cereals are made from one of three ingredients: oats, rice or wheat. Each of these core ingredients has a number of nutritional benefits. Oats, for example, are thought to help lower cholesterol as part of a healthy diet, while wheat is an excellent source of fibre. However, the processing techniques used in the mass production of cereals are not good for the grains. Once they have been cooked, conditioned, flattened, toasted and shredded, much of their nutritional value – and flavour – is lost. The flavour will be replaced with salt, "frosted" sugar or a glaze of syrup, while the lost nutrients are restored as "added vitamins and minerals", which can then be promoted on the box.

The level of processing involved in the production of cereal means that there is room for countless variations on the standard formula. The addition of nuts, berries, or honey to a simple cereal adds novelty value, but a better nutritional option may be to buy an unadorned version (which will almost always be lower in sugar and fat) and add your own toppings at home.

HEALTH CLAIMS

Given the production techniques described above, the number of health claims ascribed to popular breakfast foods might come as something of a surprise. Often, the addition of vitamins and minerals creates a halo of healthiness around a product that is actually high in salt, sugar and fat. Fortified products can be useful, but are not a substitute for a balanced diet: a fortified cereal that offers 2mg of iron per serving actually contains no more iron than two slices of (unfortified) wholemeal bread – and the bread is much less likely to be high in fat.

One health claim that has been officially sanctioned is the link between wholegrain and heart health. Manufacturers of products that contain at least 50 per cent whole grain by weight are allowed to label their products with a statement such as "whole-grains can help keep the heart healthy as part of a balanced diet". However, the phrase "contains wholegrain" now appears on a wide range of cereals – some of which, inevitably, are also high in ingredients that are anything but good for the heart.

MORE SUGAR THAN A JAM DOUGHNUT

The Advertising Standards Authority, when it upheld a claim against a 2004 campaign for Frosties, noted that a bowl of the product with 125ml of milk contained more sugar than a jam doughnut. It appears that this is not unusual; the situation has become so bad that consumer magazine Which? has singled out breakfast cereals as the target of a campaign against the misleading promotion of high fat, salt and sugar (HFSS) foods. There are particular concerns about the targeting of these products at children, as successive studies have shown that children's cereals tend to be amongst the highest in added sugar.

One of the most heavily criticised innovations is the biscuit straw, advertised by its two main manufacturers, Kellogg's and Nestlé, as a way of encouraging children to drink milk. The straws, made from a wheat biscuit coated in chocolate, have been described in terms of their sugar content as the equivalent of a KitKat, something few parents would choose to give their children for breakfast.

Cereals aimed at adults can also be unexpectedly sweet. Some dried fruit mueslis are sweetened twice, once in the oats and a second time in the preserved fruits. Others, especially plain bran cereals, can contain high levels of salt. This is particularly worrying when the products are being sold on the basis of their health credentials as a good source of fibre.

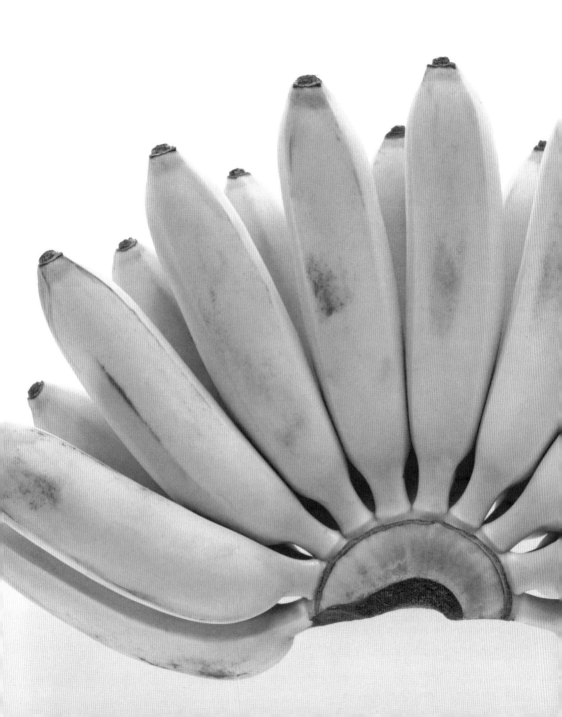

OUR RESEARCH RESULTS

The most striking aspect of the Breakfast Cereals table is the diversity of results on offer. In each of the four categories there is an almost haphazard selection of red, amber and green lights, with high sugars, fats and salt jostling for space with their exact opposites – sometimes in the same column. Frosties, for instance, have been the subject of much criticism for their high sugar content, but also have the lowest saturated fats of any cereal in the table – including "heart healthy" products such as oats and wheat. This, amongst other surprises, suggests that cereals is one product category in which every single result counts.

As expected, the majority of the cereals surveyed receive a red light for sugar, with Kellogg's Frosties and Coco Pops leading the table at 37 and 36g per 100g respectively. By way of comparison, 100g of Green & Black's 70% dark chocolate contains only 29.4g of sugars. Unlike chocolate, however, both of these products are relatively low in fat. By far the fattiest product on offer is Jordans Original Crunchy Tropical Fruits, with 14.5g per 100g. Jordans is also the only product in the table to get a red light for saturates. It does, however, contain just a trace of salt. Kellogg's Corn Flakes and Nestlé Cinnamon Grahams, on the other hand, have 1.8g of salt per 100g. But as the sole cereal with four green lights, Nestlé Shredded Wheat has the top score.

THE GOOD NUTRITION GUIDE RECOMMENDS

LOWEST IN SUGARS:
Shredded Wheat

LOWEST IN SATURATED FATS:
Frosties

LOWEST IN SALT:
Jordans Crunchy Tropical Fruits; Shredded Wheat; Sugar Puffs; Quaker Oats; Ready Brek

THE GOOD NUTRITION GUIDE BEST CHOICE:
Shredded Wheat

THE GOOD NUTRITION GUIDE WORST CHOICE:
Nestle Curiously Cinnamon

BRAND NAME	Energy	Protein	Fibre	Carbohydrates	Sugars	Fat	Saturated Fat	Salt	Good Nutrition Guide Score	Company group
Jordans Original Crunchy Tropical Fruits	423	8.1	6.7	65.1	26.3	14.5	5.1	0.0	37.5	Jordans Cereals
Kellogg's Fruit 'n Fibre	358	8	10	68	23.0	6.0	3.5	1.4	37.5	Kellogg's
Kellogg's All Bran Original	280	14	27	48	17.0	3.5	0.7	1.6	37.5	Kellogg's
Kellogg's Coco Pops	387	5	2	85	36.0	3.0	1.5	1.2	62.5	Kellogg's
Kellogg's Corn Flakes	372	7	3	84	8.0	0.9	0.2	1.8	62.5	Kellogg's
Kellogg's Crunchy Nut	397	6	2.5	82	35.0	5.0	0.9	1.2	50.0	Kellogg's
Kellogg's Frosties	371	4.5	2	87	37.0	0.6	0.1	0.2	75.0	Kellogg's
Kellogg's Rice Krispies	381	6	1	87	10.0	1.0	0.2	1.7	62.5	Kellogg's
Nestle Cheerios	368	8.1	6.5	75.1	21.6	3.9	1.1	1.2	50.0	Nestle
Nestle Curiously Cinnamon	411	4.7	4.2	76.1	34.2	9.8	3.7	1.8	25.0	Nestle
Nestle Honey Nut Cheerios	374	6.9	5.1	78.2	35.4	3.7	0.9	1.1	50.0	Nestle
Nestle Shreddies	351	9.9	9.8	73.5	15.5	1.9	0.4	0.1	62.5	Nestle
Nestle Shredded Wheat	340	11.6	11.8	67.8	0.9	2.5	0.5	0.0	100	Nestle
Sugar Puffs	379	5.3	3.7	85.8	35.0	1.6	0.2	0.0	75.0	Quaker Oats
Quaker Oats	356	11	9	60	1.1	8.0	1.5	0.0	87.5	Quaker Oats
Alpen Raisins, Hazelnuts & Almonds	359	10.5	7.3	66.6	21.8	5.8	0.7	0.4	50.0	Weetabix
Ready Brek	358	11.8	7.9	58.5	1.0	8.7	1.2	0.0	87.5	Weetabix
Weetabix	338	11.5	10	68.4	4.4	2.0	0.6	0.7	87.5	Weetabix

Key

Typical serving size: 40g (medium bowl)

All figures are grammes per 100 grammes (expect Energy reading which = Kcal per100 grammes)

Source: The Ethical Company Organisation / The Good Nutrition Guide 2006 - 2008

For explantion of Good Nutrition Guide Score see the "Using the Research Tables" section

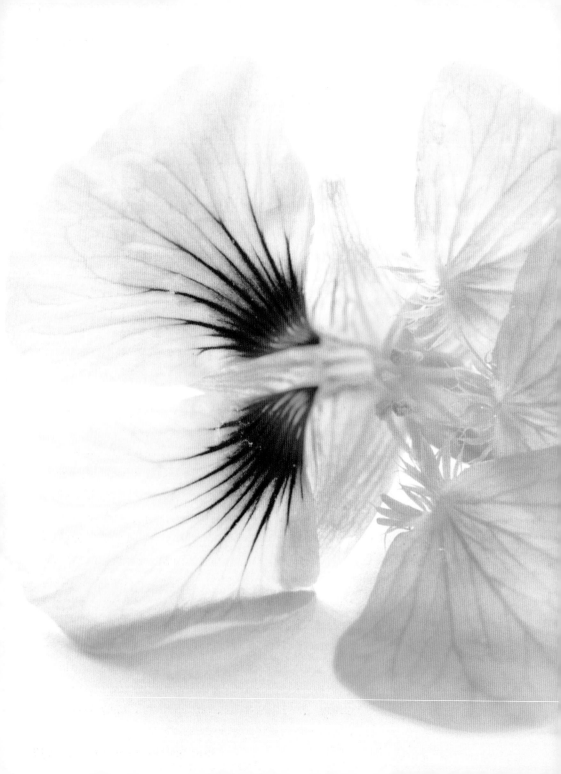

Butter and Margarine

Once upon a time fans of butter were encouraged to switch to margarine because it was believed to be better for their health. Now it appears that margarine may not be the nutritious alternative it once appeared, and reduced fat or "butter-like" spreads have largely taken its place. The choice for the health-conscious consumer is between the imitation low-fat spread, with its emulsifiers and artificial colours, the olive oil-based margarine or the occasional indulgence of the real thing. Or, for those who prefer to sit on the fence, a balanced combination of all three.

A SPREAD OF SPREADS

Pure butters contain nothing but cream, and are made by churning the fats in cows' milk until they reach a solid consistency. Some butters contain salt, so if you add salt to your foods during cooking be aware that you could be seasoning your meals twice – or three times if you also keep salt at the table. Unsalted butters are available for those who are watching their intake.

Margarines are made from a combination of ingredients. Usually 80 per cent of these will be animal, vegetable or fish oils (check the label if you are a vegetarian), while the other 20 per cent will consist of added ingredients including milk, and additives such as colourings,

flavourings and emulsifiers. Nearly all margarines are salted, and by law all are fortified with vitamins A and D. Some low fat spreads contain water, and use pork gelatine to maintain their texture.

Products that contain less than 80 per cent oils or fats must be labelled as "spreads". There are strict definitions for the labelling of "low" and "reduced fat" spreads. A "reduced fat" spread is one that contains up to 60 per cent fat. A "low fat" spread must contain less than 40 per cent fat, while a "very low fat" spread must have no more than 30 per cent fat.

Amongst the spreads are numerous "butter-like" products that emulate the texture and flavour of butter but contain less of the fat. They are usually dairy spreads with added cream or buttermilk, and invariably use extra flavourings and colourings such as annatto and curcumin to produce a more buttery appearance.

WHICH FAT IS BEST?

There is much debate over which is healthier: butter or margarine. For a long time it had been assumed that margarine was the better option because it was lower in saturated fats, but there are now concerns that the other fats in margarine may be even worse for our health. These other fats are trans fats, which have been discovered to raise the level of LDL, the "bad cholesterol" in our blood. They appear on the ingredients list as hydrogenated or partially hydrogenated oils, and are produced in the processes used to make the margarine. Some margarines are now available that do not contain trans fats – these are likely to be a better option.

Some margarines use olive oil rather than vegetable oil. Olive oil is high in monounsaturated fats, which are thought to help protect against cardiovascular disease, so the products are often sold as healthier alternatives to standard margarine. Nevertheless, olive oil products are also high in fat so should still be consumed in moderation.

THE "NUTRICEUTICALS"

"Nutriceuticals" are foods that have either been identified for their health benefits, or modified to give them properties beyond their normal nutrient content. Otherwise known as functional foods, they now include a number of brands of margarine. Many of these claim to reduce cholesterol as part of a balanced diet. Their active ingredients are plant sterol esters, which have been shown to lower the levels of cholesterol in the blood. These products are useful for people who have been diagnosed with high cholesterol.

Other approved claims include the link between omega-3 and a healthy heart. According to the Joint Health Claims Initiative, "Eating 3g weekly, or 0.45g daily, long chain omega-3 polyunsaturated fatty acids, as part of a healthy lifestyle, helps maintain heart health." This is the claim that manufacturers can use on their products. However, the JHCI advises that products high in saturated fats should not be marketed on these terms, so check

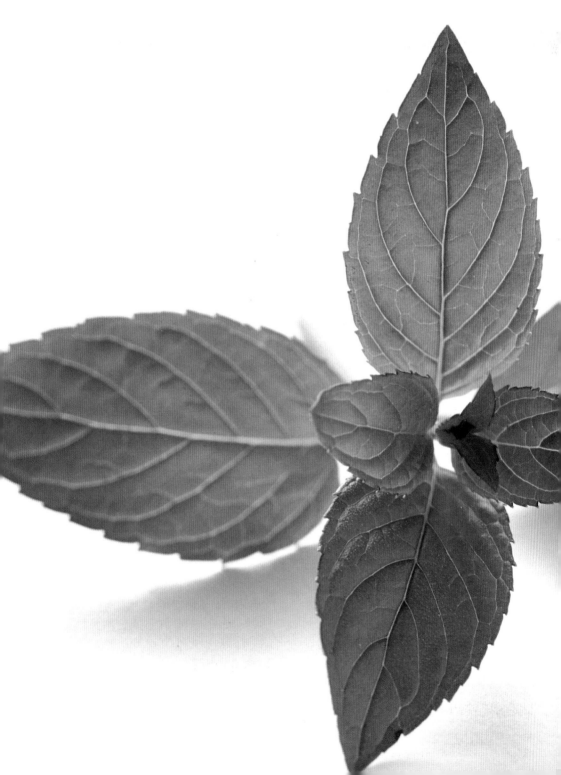

the credentials of the margarine before buying.

OUR RESEARCH RESULTS

For a product such as butter or margarine, carbohydrates and sugars are barely present: the main concerns are fats and, inevitably, hidden salt. In the case of the latter, there is a considerable difference between the highest and lowest figures. Country Life Unsalted tops the chart, and is also the only butter to get a green light for salt. Three Unilever products, Stork, Stork Spreadable and I Can't Believe It's Not Butter, list over 1.5g salt per 100g, with Stork containing the most at 2.3g.

Although its low salt figure provides Country Life with a high overall score, it also has by far the largest amount of saturated fat. At 54.7g per 100g, this product contains significantly more saturates than the second highest, Lurpak Spreadable, at 37g. It also has the most fat in total, although not by much – Anchor and Lurpak Spreadable both have 80g compared with Country Life's 82.7g. The one vegan product in the list, Pure With Soya, receives average marks for both fats and salt, but is higher in fat than the low fat products from both Flora and St Ivel. Indeed, St Ivel Gold Low Fat is the lowest in both fat and saturates, and only misses out on an overall recommendation because of its higher salt content.

THE GOOD NUTRITION GUIDE RECOMMENDS

LOWEST IN SUGARS:
Country Life Unsalted; Pure With Soya; Flora Light; Flora Original; Flora Pro. activ; Stork; Stork Spreadable

LOWEST IN SATURATED FATS:
St Ivel Gold Low Fat

LOWEST IN SALT:
Country Life Unsalted

THE GOOD NUTRITION GUIDE BEST CHOICE:
Country Life Unsalted

THE GOOD NUTRITION GUIDE WORST CHOICE:
I Can't Believe It's Not Butter; Stork; Stork Spreadable

BRAND NAME	ENERGY	PROTEIN	FIBRE	CARBOHYDRATES	SUGARS	FAT	SATURATED FAT	SALT	GOOD NUTRITION GUIDE SCORE	Company group
ANCHOR SPREADABLE	722.0	0.3	0.0	0.3	0.3	80.0	31.2	1.3	37.5	Arla Foods
LURPAK SPREADABLE SLIGHTLY SALTED	728.0	1.0	0.0	1.0	1.0	80.0	37.0	0.9	37.5	Arla Foods
COUNTRY LIFE UNSALTED	746.0	0.5	0.0	0.0	0.0	82.7	54.7	0.0	50.0	Dairy Crest
ST IVEL GOLD LOW FAT	330.0	0.5	0.0	3.1	0.7	35.0	8.7	1.5	37.5	Dairy Crest
PURE WITH SOYA	531.0	0.0	0.0	0.0	0.0	51.0	14.0	0.8	37.5	Matthews Foods
BERTOLLI OLIVE OIL SPREAD	536.0	0.2	0.0	1.0	1.0	59.0	14.0	0.8	37.5	Unilever
FLORA LIGHT	366.0	0.1	0.0	6.0	0.0	38.0	9.3	1.0	37.5	Unilever
FLORA ORIGINAL	531.0	0.0	0.0	0.0	0.0	59.0	12.0	1.4	37.5	Unilever
FLORA PRO.ACTIV	324.0	0.1	0.0	2.5	0.0	35.0	9.0	1.0	37.5	Unilever
I CAN'T BELIEVE IT'S NOT BUTTER	635.0	0.5	0.0	0.7	0.7	70.0	25.7	1.7	25.0	Unilever
STORK	675.0	0.0	0.0	0.0	0.0	75.0	27.4	2.3	25.0	Unilever
STORK SPREADABLE	531.0	0.0	0.0	0.0	0.0	59.0	21.0	1.7	25.0	Unilever

Key

TYPICAL SERVING SIZE: 10G (two teaspoons)

All figures are grammes per 100 grammes (expect Energy reading which = Kcal per100 grammes)

Source: The Ethical Company Organisation / The Good Nutrition Guide 2006 - 2008

For explantion of Good Nutrition Guide Score see the "Using the Research Tables" section

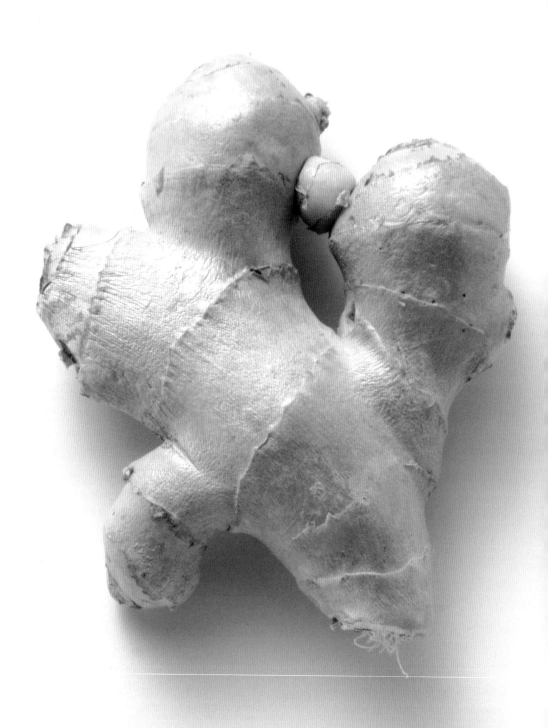

Cakes

Even the most cursory glance at the nutrition panel will reveal that cake is not a particularly nutritious substance, and shop-bought cakes – which are often laden with additives as well as the usual fat and sugar – are amongst the worst. This makes recommending the healthy option a little tricky, although there are always alternatives that are slightly lower in saturated fat or higher in fibre, and these are often worth considering. Unfortunately, despite the best efforts of modern science, the fabled healthy cake remains elusive.

THE "HEALTHY EATING" OPTION

Under the Food Standards Agency's traffic light labelling system, most cakes will earn three red lights for fat, saturates and sugar. This doesn't bode well for their nutritional value, but it is possible to find varieties that are lower in the ingredients that are least beneficial to health. Perhaps the most important nutrient to limit is saturated fat, which has been shown to increase the risk of cardiovascular disease in later life.

Often, the best choices are not the "healthy eating" options. Many of these focus on reducing one particular ingredient – for example, by replacing sugar with sweeteners – whilst ignoring others that can be equally damaging. Inevitably, the feel-good factor of buying a "better" product makes many of us less inclined to refuse second helpings. Be aware that if a mainstream company launches its own healthy range, the claims relate only to other products in the line: their "reduced fat" cake may be just as fatty as the standard version from another company.

In general, cakes with icing or cream centres are likely to contain more sugar (and more calories) than those without. Despite the nutritional appeal of real fruit, most traditional fruit cakes owe their longevity to vast quantities of molasses – although mass-produced, sponge-based varieties may be less sugary. Brightly coloured cakes and children's products will usually be high in artificial colours and flavourings, some of which could cause allergic reactions in susceptible individuals.

Flapjacks are easy to mistake for a healthy sweet treat, but don't be fooled by the presence of cholesterol-lowering oats: in terms of their sugar and fat content, these are simply cakes in disguise. Nevertheless, flapjacks and cakes made with wholemeal flour can at least boast a slightly higher fibre content.

A PIECE OF CAKE

Working out the size of a piece of cake is not, to use an old phrase, a piece of cake. How wide is a single slice of cake? Is one small cake equal to a portion of a big cake? Does a sliver of Swiss roll compare with a jam tart? Looking at the figures per 100g may give you a better idea of how they measure up, but it is not always possible to compare like with like. When in doubt, check what the box lists as a recommended serving – it may be less than you expect.

Indeed, by dividing their packets into individually wrapped pairs, some companies encourage the consumption of two cakes per sitting (because there's no point letting one of them go stale...) even though their recommended serving is only one. If this is the case, don't forget to double the nutritional information figures to find out how much you're really eating.

TRANS FATS

As well as the better known saturates, cakes can also be a source of trans fats. These are produced during the hydrogenation of oils, meaning that if a label lists "hydrogenated vegetable oil", the chances are the product contains trans fats. At the moment trans fats do not have to be labelled separately on nutrition panels in the UK, so they will only appear as part of the total figure for fats. There is increasing pressure on companies to reveal the trans fat content of their foods, and one cake manufacturer – Mr Kipling – is leading the way by including separate figures for trans fats on its website.

Instead of using oil from vegetable sources, some cakes use animal fats. This means that they are not suitable for vegetarians; guidance will be given on the label.

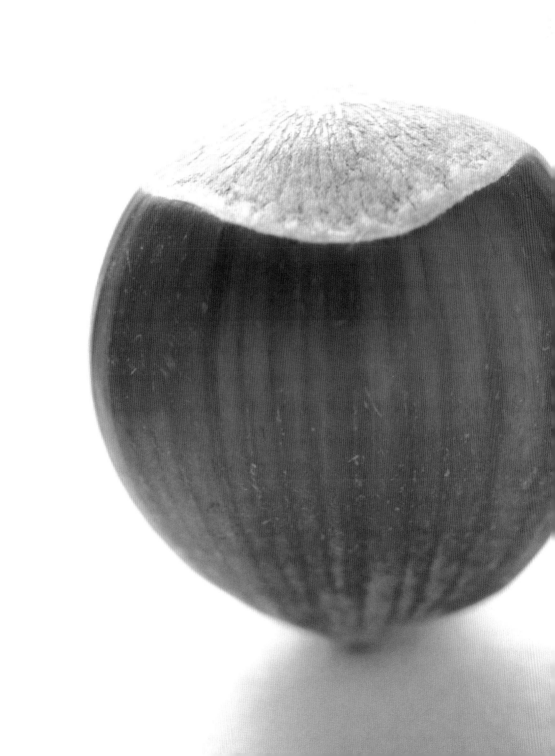

Our Research Results

As expected, the Cakes table is full of high fat, high sugar products. Nevertheless, there is still enough scope between the different brands to make an informed nutritional choice worthwhile. Starting with sugars, there is a range of over 30g between the highest and lowest figures in the survey. By a slim margin, Mr Kipling Apple Pies contain the least sugar at 28.8g per 100g. With 59.4g per 100g, Mr Kipling French Fancies have the most. Clearly, variation is as common between different types of product as it is between different brands.

This is certainly true of fat and saturates levels. Here, only three products receive a red light for fat, with Fabulous Bakin' Boys Chocolate Cup Cakes and Thorntons Toffee Cakes both appearing particularly high in this nutrient. By far the lowest in fat are WeightWatchers Chocolate Brownies, which are also the only cakes in the table to get a green light for saturates. Thorntons Toffee Cakes cement their reputation as an indulgence with a huge 14.1g saturates per 100g. Mr Kipling's Battenburg and French Fancies, although high in sugars, are relatively low in saturates.

Salt inevitably makes an appearance in many of these sweet products: Fabulous Bakin' Boys Chocolate Cup Cakes and McVitie's Lyle's Golden Syrup Cake both contain a gram of salt per 100g. Two Mr Kipling items, Apple Pies and Cherry Bakewells, are the least salty at 0.3g per 100g. With the lowest calorie level overall, WeightWatchers Chocolate Brownies live up to their name as a low cal, low fat option.

The Good Nutrition Guide Recommends

Lowest in Sugars:
Mr Kipling Apple Pies

Lowest in Saturated Fats:
WeightWatchers Chocolate Brownies

Lowest in Salt:
Mr Kipling Apple Pies; Mr Kipling Cherry Bakewells

Best Choice:
WeightWatchers Chocolate Brownies

BRAND NAME	ENERGY	PROTEIN	FIBRE	CARBOHYDRATES	SUGARS	FAT	SATURATED FAT	SALT	GOOD NUTRITION GUIDE SCORE	Company group
WEIGHTWATCHERS CHOCOLATE BROWNIES	304.0	4.8	3.2	62.5	48.9	3.8	1.3	0.4	50.0	Anthony Alan Foods
FABULOUS BAKIN' BOYS CHOCOLATE CUP CAKES	432.0	4.0	3.0	54.0	32.0	24.0	8.0	1.0	12.5	Fabulous Bakin' Boys
MR KIPLING FRENCH FANCIES	369.0	2.8	0.6	68.3	59.4	9.4	3.7	0.8	37.5	Kipling Cakes
MR KIPLING APPLE PIES	350.0	3.5	1.3	53.5	28.8	13.6	5.1	0.3	37.5	Kipling Cakes
MR KIPLING BATTENBERG	416.0	6.1	1.3	70.5	55.9	12.2	3.9	0.5	37.5	Kipling Cakes
MR KIPLING CHERRY BAKEWELLS	428.0	3.9	1.4	61.3	40.2	18.5	8.5	0.3	37.5	Kipling Cakes
MR KIPLING VICTORIA SLICES	430.0	4.0	1.2	68.2	43.3	15.6	9.3	0.8	25.0	Kipling Cakes
MCVITIE'S LYLE'S GOLDEN SYRUP CAKE	355.0	3.4	1.4	60.4	39.1	11.0	3.4	1.0	37.5	McVitie's / Tate & Lyle
THORNTONS TOFFEE CAKES	476.0	4.5	2.1	54.5	40.5	26.7	14.1	0.4	12.5	Thorntons
MCVITIE'S HOBNOB FLAPJACKS	447.0	5.7	0.7	59.2	29.2	20.9	9.3	0.8	12.5	United Biscuits

Key

TYPICAL SERVING SIZE: 70G (single slice / mini pie)
All figures are grammes per 100 grammes (expect Energy reading which = Kcal per100 grammes)
Source: The Ethical Company Organisation / The Good Nutrition Guide 2006 - 2008
For explantion of Good Nutrition Guide Score see the "Using the Research Tables" section

WORST CHOICE:

Fabulous Bakin' Boys Chocolate Cup
Cakes; Thorntons Toffee Cakes; McVitie's
HobNob Flapjacks

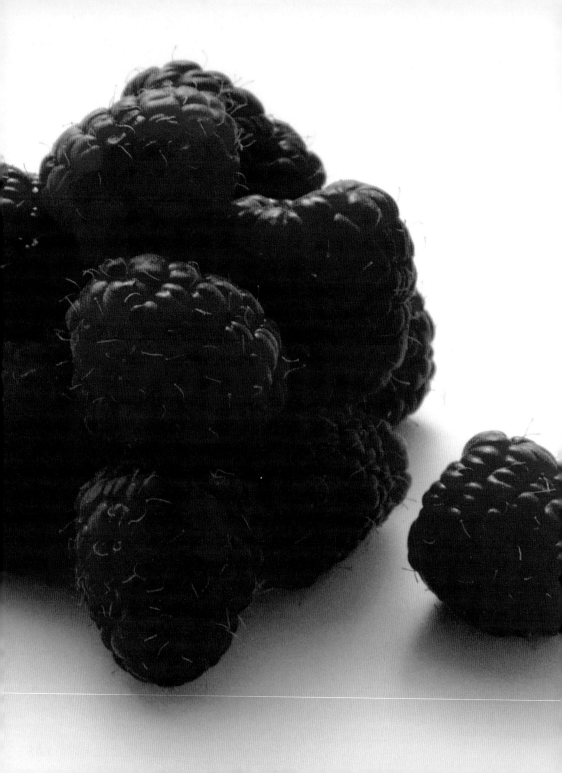

Cereal Bars

Cereal manufacturers would like us to believe that their products are not merely a breakfast item but a healthy snack at any time of the day. Nowhere is this clearer than in the invention of the breakfast bar – essentially a bowl of cereal in biscuit form. As food on the go, cereal bars seem ideal for those who might otherwise skip breakfast, but in some cases they are no more nutritious than an actual biscuit. High in sugar and fat, cereal bars are not always a healthy start to the day.

A Good Breakfast

As the meal that breaks our night-time fast, breakfast is arguably the most important meal of the day. People who don't have a proper breakfast are more likely to snack, and less likely to have stable energy levels in the morning. Studies have also indicated that breakfast can have a positive effect on cognitive function, so it is particularly important that children have something to eat before going to school.

Breakfast bars may encourage us to eat breakfast, but they also facilitate the belief that this important meal can be reduced to a snack: imagine the outcry if it was suggested that we could replace lunch in a similar way. The key question, then, is whether or not cereal bars provide a nutritionally balanced alternative to a full breakfast.

Nutritional Content

To get an idea of how the nutritional content of a cereal changes when it is made into a cereal bar, have a look at the ingredients lists for Kellogg's original Special K cereal and their Special K cereal bars:

Special K contains:

Rice, Wheat (Wholewheat, Wheat Flour), Sugar, Wheat Gluten, Dried Skimmed Milk, Salt, Defatted Wheatgerm, Barley Malt Flavouring, Vitamin C, Niacin, Iron, Vitamin B6, Riboflavin (B2), Thiamin (B1), Folic Acid, Vitamin D, Vitamin B12.

Special K cereal bar contains:

Kellogg's Special K Cereal (43%) (Rice, Wheat {Wholewheat, Wheat Flour}, Sugar, Wheat Gluten, Dried Skimmed Milk, Salt, Defatted Wheatgerm, Barley Malt Flavouring, Vitamin C, Niacin, Iron, Vitamin B6, Riboflavin (B2), Thiamin (B1), Folic Acid, Vitamin B12), Glucose Syrup, Strawberry Flavour Fruit Pieces (8%)(Sugar, Cranberries, Citric Acid, Strawberry Flavouring, Elderberry Juice Concentrate), Sugar, Fructose, Hydrogenated Vegetable Oil, Dextrose, Dried Skimmed Milk, Humectant (Sorbitol, Glycerol), Milk Fat, Calcium Carbonate, Milk Sugar, Flavourings, Emulsifier (Soy Lecithin), Antioxidant (E320).

As well as all the ingredients of Special K, the cereal bar also contains five separate types of sugar (glucose syrup, sugar, fructose, dextrose and milk sugar), flavourings, emulsifiers, antioxidants and hydrogenated vegetable oil, a source of potentially damaging trans fats.

Added Vitamins and Minerals

The claim of "added vitamins and minerals" that appears on many breakfast bar packets may not be as impressive as it seems. To use the example given above, the amount of added vitamins in the cereal bar is far less than in the original cereal – not surprising as the bar is only 43 per cent Special K. The only mineral for which cereal bars are likely to improve on their dry cereal counterparts is iron, although this is mostly because they already contain milk.

Another popular added mineral is calcium, which is crucial in the development of healthy teeth and bones. Nevertheless, it's worth remembering that a serving of one-third of a pint of semi skimmed milk on a bowl of cereal contains 230mg calcium – significantly more than in the average breakfast bar. For all these claims, the best advice is to check them thoroughly. If this is impractical, base your purchases on other significant factors (such as low levels of added sugar) rather than any particular health claim.

When is a Cereal Bar Not a Cereal Bar?

The more the cereal bar market has grown, the more difficult it has become to distinguish between "breakfast products" and simple "snacks", particularly if

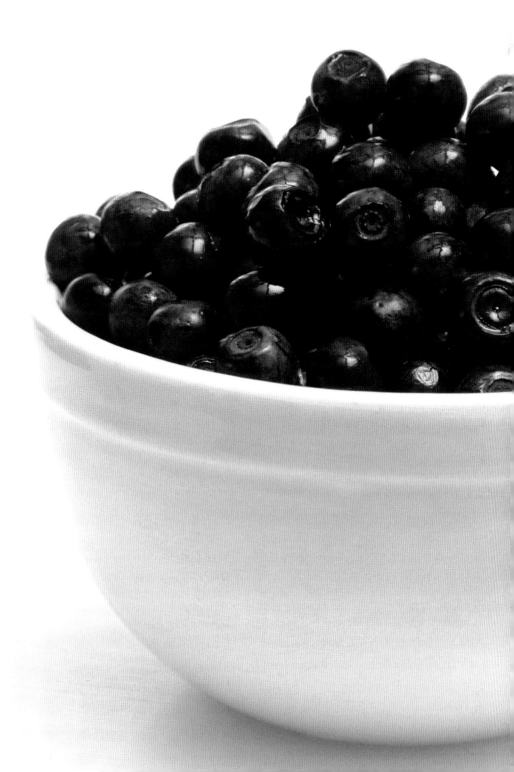

they are found alongside each other on the supermarket shelf. Often the key nutritional values are not that different: for example, Nestlé's Nesquik Bar contains more saturated fat per serving than one of Kellogg's "Crazy Choc" Rice Krispies Squares, even though the former is a fortified breakfast bar and the latter is a snack.

OUR RESEARCH RESULTS

Despite their smaller serving sizes, cereal bars do not compare particularly well with breakfast cereals when it comes to high levels of sugar and fat. From the table it appears that cereal bars are, on average, even more sugary than breakfast cereals. Three cereal bars (Cadbury Raisin Brunch Bar, Traidcraft Geobar Raisin & Apricot and Weetos Bars) contain more than 40g of sugars per 100g, compared with none of the breakfast cereals surveyed; every single cereal bar receives a red light for sugar.

All of the cereal bars, with the exception of Ryvita's Apple and Sultana Goodness Bars, receive amber or red lights for fats. Only the Tracker Choc Chip has two red lights for fats and saturates, but many products – including Cadbury Raisin

Brunch Bar and Harvest Chewee Milk Choc Chip Cereal Bar – contain over 5g of saturates. While a distinction should be made between snack bars such as the Cadbury product and "breakfast" bars, the bars based on popular cereals generally fare little better. The Nestlé Fitnesse Cereal Bar (based on a low-fat cereal) contains 7.0g fat and 3.9g saturates per 100g – less than many products in the table, but still a substantial amount compared with the 99% fat free cereal. The Special K bar is the saltiest in the survey, with 1g salt per 100g. Only the Jordans and Ryvita bars contain no salt at all.

Overall, these figures suggest that while there is plenty to choose from between the big name cereals, there are few real alternatives amongst their related cereal bars. If you are looking for a wide selection of low sugar, low fat breakfast bars, you may be disappointed.

THE GOOD SHOPPING GUIDE RECOMMENDS

LOWEST IN SUGARS:
Quaker Oat Bar

LOWEST IN SATURATED FATS:
Ryvita Apple & Sultana Goodness Bars

Brand Name	Energy	Protein	Fibre	Carbohydrates	Sugars	Fat	Saturated Fat	Salt	Good Nutrition Guide Score	Company group
Cadbury Raisin Brunch Bar	430.0	5.6	1.8	66.4	42.2	15.5	7.9	0.6	25.0	Cadbury Schweppes
Nature Valley Crunchy Granola Oat & Honey	445.0	8.3	6.2	70.4	27.0	16.1	2.0	0.9	37.5	General Mills
Jordans Wild Berries Frusli Bars	392.0	5.7	5.0	70.0	30.8	9.9	2.1	0.0	50.0	Jordans Cereals
Kellogg's Nutrigrain Soft Bake Bars	355.0	4.0	4.0	67.0	32.0	9.0	3.5	0.8	37.5	Kellogg's
Kellogg's Rice Krispie Squares	406.0	3.0	0.9	72.0	32.0	12.0	5.0	0.8	37.5	Kellogg's
Special K Original	400.0	8.0	2.0	75.0	35.0	8.0	3.0	1.0	37.5	Kellogg's
Tracker Choc Chip	488.0	6.8	1.9	59.2	29.8	23.7	12.0	0.5	12.5	Masterfoods
Nestle Fitnesse Cereal Bar	382.0	5.1	3.2	74.8	30.1	7.0	3.9	0.8	37.5	Nestle
Harvest Chewee Milk Choc Chip Cereal Bar	430.0	5.5	3.5	68.0	29.0	16.0	7.2	0.5	25.0	Quaker Oats
Quaker Oat Bar	366.0	7.2	8.0	64.4	16.7	9.4	2.5	0.5	37.5	Quaker Oats
Ryvita Apple & Sultana Goodness Bars	268.0	4.3	22.0	56.4	24.3	2.8	0.4	0.0	75.0	Ryvita Company
Traidcraft Geobar Raisin & Apricot	377.0	4.4	3.0	71.2	42.2	8.3	6.0	0.2	37.5	Traidcraft
Alpen Fruit & Nut Bars	394.0	6.5	4.6	71.2	29.5	9.2	2.9	0.5	37.5	Weetabix
Weetos Bars	440.0	5.9	1.6	70.9	40.9	14.7	7.2	0.3	37.5	Weetabix

Key

Typical serving size: 100g (two scoops)

All figures are grammes per 100 grammes (expect Energy reading which = Kcal per100 grammes)

Source: The Ethical Company Organisation / The Good Nutrition Guide 2006 - 2008

For explantion of Good Nutrition Guide Score see the "Using the Research Tables" section

Lowest in Salt:

Jordans Wild Berries Frusli Bars; Ryvita Apple & Sultana Goodness Bars

The Good Nutrition Guide
Best Choice:

Ryvita Apple & Sultana Goodness Bars

The Good Nutrition Guide
Worst Choice:

Tracker Choc Chip

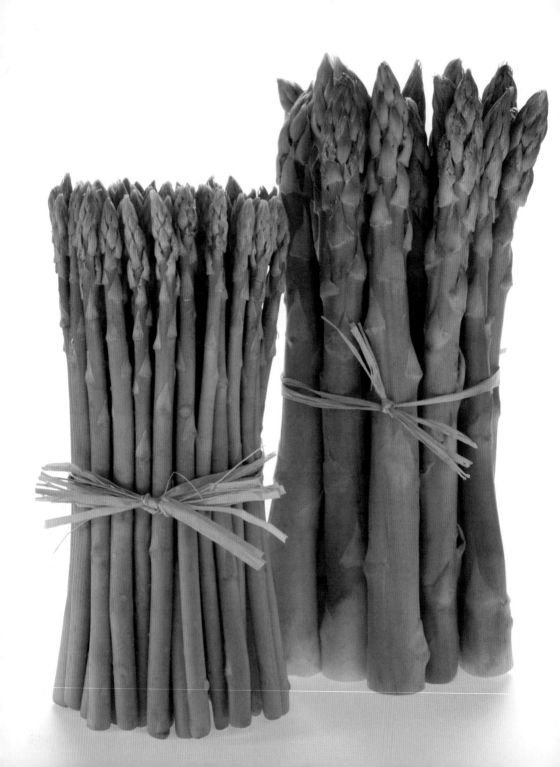

Cheese

It used to be that you could tell where you were in the world by the dairy products on offer, from Parmesan in Italy to cheddar in Cheddar. Now even the smallest supermarkets stock a cornucopia of cheeses from right across the globe. While it would be easy to assume that cheese is essentially cheese (it's all made from milk, after all) there is a surprising amount of nutritional variation on offer. This is particularly true of some processed cheeses, which many would argue stretch the definition of "cheese" as far as it will go.

CURDS AND WHEY

Cheese is made from milk that has been separated into curds (solids) and whey (the remaining liquids) by the enzymes in a substance called rennet. Rennet is found in the stomachs of animals such as cows, where it acts as a digestive aid, although many manufacturers now derive their rennet from vegetarian sources – check the label to be sure.

Varieties of cheese such as cheddar, brie and stilton obtain their distinctive flavours and textures from the bacteria and moulds that act upon the milk. Other types are produced by the addition of herbs, or by varying the kind of milk and its fat content. The lower the moisture level in a cheese, the harder it will be.

A common criticism of supermarket cheese is that it is not given enough time to properly mature. Cheeses are traditionally kept at much higher temperatures than those in supermarket refrigeration units in order to allow the bacteria to flourish; as far as the big stores are concerned, this would be a health and safety hazard. Many cheeses have their flavours enhanced with other ingredients – such as fruits and spices – rather than being allowed to ripen of their own accord.

DAIRY PRODUCTS

Dairy products such as cheese are important in a balanced diet as they provide a good source of calcium and other vitamins and minerals such as phosphorus. They are also an efficient source of protein: it takes approximately 10 litres of milk to make 1kg of cheese. However, cheeses – like all dairy products – can be high in fat, so should be consumed in moderation. For those on a lower dairy intake, calcium can be obtained from non-dairy foods including sardines, soya and tofu, beans and green vegetables.

Many of the most popular cheeses are available in low-fat versions, but check the label to see if the reduction is significant compared to other brands. Further low fat options include cottage cheese and reduced-fat cream cheeses. There is little difference in fat content between cows' and goats' milk, although hard goats' cheeses usually fall in the high fat range. As with other products, watch out for saturates as well as the overall fat content.

PROCESSED CHEESE

Processed cheeses are cheeses that have been modified, usually with the addition of emulsifiers and colourings, to give them a longer shelf-life and make them suitable for individual wrapping. They are usually packaged in squares or triangles, although

one American company has taken the novel approach of selling theirs in a spray can. Some of these "cheeses" contain very little actual cheese, so are required by law to be labelled as a "product", "food" or "spread". When this is the case, the cheese will often be bulked up with milk.

SALT

The Food Standards Agency lists cheese as one of its "foods that are often high in salt". These are foods that, as a matter of course, contain significant amounts of sodium (more than 0.5g per 100g). Although all cheeses are salty, there are still significant differences between the various brands and categories. Processed cheese products – particularly the cheese slices and triangles that appeal to children – tend to be especially salty.

OUR RESEARCH RESULTS

While it would be easy to assume that the key nutrients of concern in this table are fats and salt, in fact the row for sugars is by far the most telling. Cheese is not by nature a sugary food, but some of the products surveyed have nevertheless

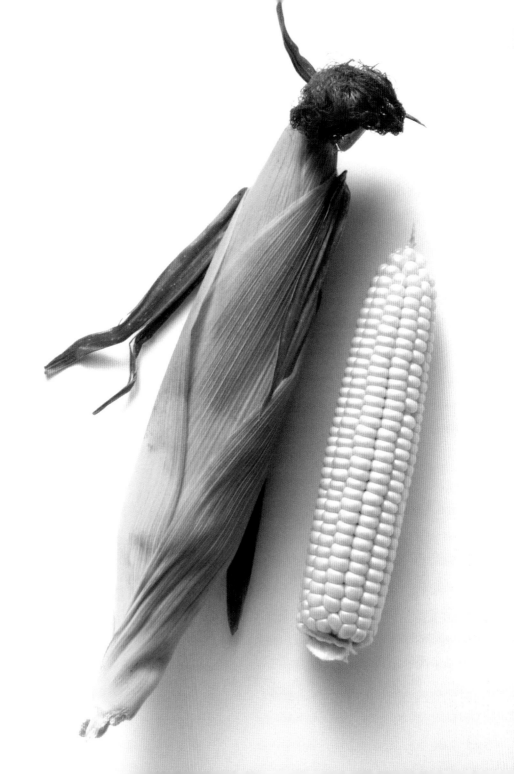

received an amber light in this category. All products in the Kraft Dairylea range contain more than 5g of sugars, while the two Laughing Cow products both contain over 6g per 100g. High sugars suggest that a cheese is likely to have been made from milk powder, meaning that it has been processed rather than matured using traditional techniques.

Accordingly, these products tend to be lower in fat, although some – such as The Laughing Cow Cheese Spread, still contain significant amounts of saturates. Discover Creamy Blue is highest in both fats and saturates overall with 37g fats per 100g, closely followed by Cathedral City Mature Cheddar at 34.9g. Lowest is The Laughing Cow Light Cheese Spread, with over half the fat (7g) of its standard equivalent. Also useful are the protein figures, which reveal that Philadelphia contains a mere 5.9g, in comparison with Cheesestrings, Cathedral City and many others at over 25g per 100g.

Regular eaters of cheese may also be surprised by the amount of salt their favourite biscuit accompaniment contains. Highest of all is Rosenborg Danish Blue with 3.8g per 100g, followed by Apetina Feta at 3.3g. Of the remaining products, the majority have 1.7g salt or over per 100g. Even the least salty, Arla's Organic Light Soft Cheese, still has 0.8g per 100g. With low calories, fats and saturates (and, notably, relatively low sugars) WeightWatchers Low Fat Soft Cheese comes out on top – despite having a salt value of 3g per 100g.

THE GOOD NUTRITION GUIDE RECOMMENDS

LOWEST IN SUGARS:
Apetina Feta; Discover Creamy Blue; Colliers Powerful Welsh Cheddar; Black Peppercorn Mature Cheddar; Isle of Man Mature Cheddar; Cheesestrings

LOWEST IN SATURATED FATS:
Weightwatchers Low Fat Soft Cheese

LOWEST IN SALT:
Arla Organic Light Soft Cheese

THE GOOD NUTRITION GUIDE BEST CHOICE:
Weightwatchers Low Fat Soft Cheese

THE GOOD NUTRITION GUIDE WORST CHOICE:
Dairylea Slices

Brand Name	Energy	Protein	Fibre	Carbohydrates	Sugars	Fat	Saturated Fat	Salt	Good Nutrition Guide Score	Company group
Apetina Feta	306.0	17.0	0.0	1.0	0.0	26.0	17.0	3.3	25.0	Arla
Discover Creamy Blue	401.0	17.0	0.0	0.1	0.0	37.0	23.6	2.3	25.0	Arla
Organic Light Soft Cheese	199.0	11.0	0.0	5.0	5.0	15.0	9.6	0.8	50.0	Arla
Rosenborg Danish Blue	341.0	20.2	0.0	0.7	0.7	28.6	18.2	3.8	25.0	Arla
Xtreme Cheddar	410.0	25.5	0.0	0.1	0.1	34.4	21.7	1.8	25.0	Breeo Foods
Cathedral City Mature Cheddar	416.0	25.4	0.0	0.1	0.1	34.9	21.7	1.8	25.0	Dairy Crest
Colliers Powerful Welsh Cheddar	410.0	25.0	0.0	0.1	0.0	34.4	22.7	1.7	25.0	Fayrfields Foods
The Laughing Cow Cheese Spread	239.0	11.0	0.0	6.0	6.0	19.0	13.0	1.8	25.0	Fromageries Bel
The Laughing Cow Light Cheese Spread	141.0	13.0	0.0	6.5	6.5	7.0	4.5	2.0	37.5	Fromageries Bel
Horlick Farms Mature Cheddar	412.0	25.5	0.0	0.1	0.1	34.4	21.7	1.8	25.0	Horlick Farms & Dairys Ltd
Black Peppercorn Mature Cheddar	412.0	25.2	0.0	0.1	0.0	33.4	19.7	1.7	25.0	Isle of Man Marketing Association
Isle of Man Mature Cheddar	412.0	25.5	0.0	0.1	0.0	33.4	19.7	1.7	25.0	Isle of Man Marketing Association
Primula Cheese Spread	226.0	11.7	0.8	5.0	3.1	17.7	12.1	0.9	50.0	Kavli
WeightWatchers Low Fat Soft Cheese	112.0	18.1	1.2	3.4	1.1	2.9	2.2	3.0	62.5	Kavli
Cheesestrings	328.0	28.0	0.0	0.0	0.0	24.0	14.8	2.0	25.0	Kerry Foods
Brunchettas With Red Pepper & Onion	296.0	14.6	1.3	17.0	5.1	19.0	10.8	1.5	37.5	Kerry Foods
Dairylea Dunkers	255.0	3.2	0.8	26.0	7.1	12.5	6.9	1.5	37.5	Kraft
Dairylea Slices	275.0	13.0	0.0	8.6	7.3	21.0	13.5	2.3	12.5	Kraft
Dairyleas Spread	240.0	11.0	0.0	5.3	5.3	19.5	13.0	2.3	25.0	Kraft
Kraft Single Slices	260.0	14.0	0.0	7.6	6.4	18.5	11.0	3.3	25.0	Kraft
Philadelphia	250.0	5.9	0.2	3.2	3.2	24.0	16.0	1.0	37.5	Kraft
Philadelphia Light with Chives	160.0	8.4	0.5	4.2	4.2	12.0	7.8	1.3	50.0	Kraft
Kraft Cracker Barral Cheddar	395.0	26.0	0.0	0.1	0.1	32.0	22.0	1.8	25.0	Kraft Foods
McLelland Seriously Strong Cheddar	410.0	25.0	0.0	0.1	0.1	34.4	21.7	1.8	25.0	Lactalis McLelland
McLelland Seriously Strong Red Cheddar	410.0	24.0	0.0	0.1	0.1	34.4	21.7	1.8	25.0	Lactalis McLelland
Charlie Cheese	412.0	25.5	0.0	0.1	0.1	34.4	21.7	1.7	25.0	Singletons Dairy
St Helens Farm Goats Cheese	370.0	24.0	0.0	0.5	0.5	30.2	18.2	1.8	25.0	St Helens Farm Company
Boursin Light Ail & Fine Herbs	140.0	12.0	0.0	2.5	2.5	9.0	6.0	1.5	50.0	Unilever

Key

Typical serving size: 30-50g

All figures are grammes per 100 grammes (expect Energy reading which = Kcal per100 grammes)

Source: The Ethical Company Organisation / The Good Nutrition Guide 2006 - 2008

For explantion of Good Nutrition Guide Score see the "Using the Research Tables" section

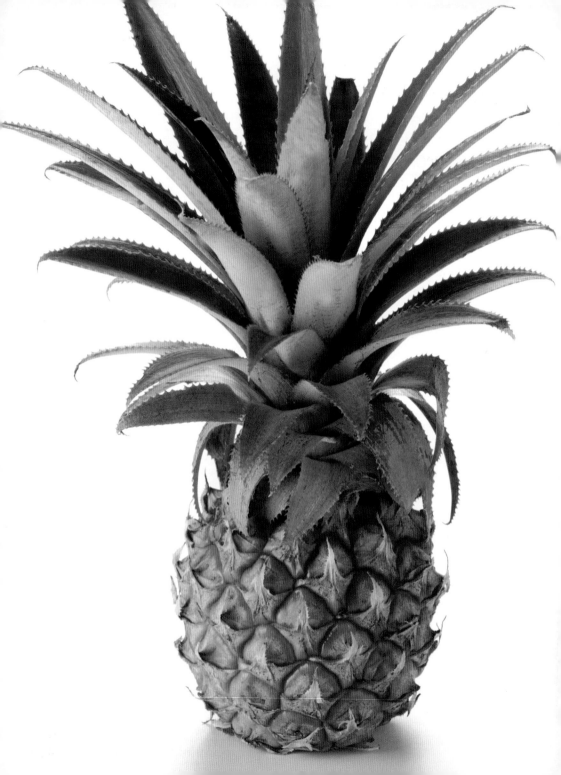

Cheese Biscuits

Fish and chips, Morecambe and Wise, cheese and crackers: some things just go together. "Biscuits for cheese" used to mean plain old cream crackers, but now it can include oatcakes, crispbreads, rice cakes and even actual biscuits. To get the most out of this age-old pairing, look for a cracker made from wholegrain, oats or rye, with minimal added salt or sugar, low levels of fat and saturates, and plenty of fibre. Avoid the "snack crackers" if possible – and keep the real biscuits for a special occasion.

CRACKERS

The simplest crackers are savoury biscuits made from wheat and yeast, often with added salt or other flavourings such as herbs. Nutritionally, the ones that are high in carbohydrate but low in sugars are a good option, as these will provide plenty of their energy from starches.

20g of fat or more per 100g is classified as a lot, and you might be shocked to find that some crackers and oatcakes (particularly those made with butter or oil) fall into this category. Others contain virtually no fat at all, so choosing one product over another can have a significant impact on what you're eating.

Salt content is crucial when it comes to crackers, partly because they are usually eaten with cheese – another foodstuff that is high in hidden salt. Generally, products that include added flavourings such as cheese powder are likely to contain more sodium, although some will also make it clear on the packet that they are a "salted" or "lightly salted" product.

CRISPBREADS, OATCAKES AND RICECAKES

Crispbreads made with wholegrain flour and no added oils will be much lower in fat and saturates than traditional crackers. Wholegrain products use the outside layers of the grain as well as the inside, which means that they are higher in fibre – an important nutrient for a healthy digestive system. As crispbreads can be slightly plain, most manufacturers use some added salt.

Oatcakes are a wheat-free alternative to crackers, and are made with wholegrain oats, usually bound together with butter or vegetable oil. As a result of this production method they can often be unexpectedly high in fat. While they rarely contain as much fibre as crispbreads, oats are naturally high in fibre, so any product listing them as the main ingredient should be a good source. Interestingly, in the Nairns range, the organic option is by far the highest in fibre. Although most of the popular oatcake brands contain no artificial additives, some do use sugar as a sweetener.

Rice cakes are a new product to infiltrate the cheese biscuit category. At their simplest, these are made from puffed rice and nothing else, but be warned: the flavoured versions are not always the saintly foods they might appear. Quaker's caramel Snack-A-Jacks, for example, may be low in fat, but they also contain a hefty 28g of sugar per 100g.

SAVOURY SNACKS

There is a fine line between cheese biscuits and just biscuits. Some types – such as Hovis Biscuits, a type of sweet digestive that often appears in selection boxes – sit on the line between the two. In nutritional terms the distinction can make a big difference. While oatcakes and crispbreads are relatively low in salt and saturated fat, some cheese snacks are more akin to crisps than crackers.

Generally, biscuits that are already flavoured with cheese, and those sold in "bite-size" portions, are more likely to fall into the snack product category than those eaten with an additional topping. Other examples of snack foods in this range include sandwich biscuits that contain a layer of cream cheese between two flavoured crackers. Crucially, the difference between "flavour" and "flavoured" is not just semantic: a cheese flavoured product will contain real cheese, while a product that lists cheese "flavour" will contain none at all. In the case of the former, the product may be a reasonable source of protein; the latter will probably be full of additives.

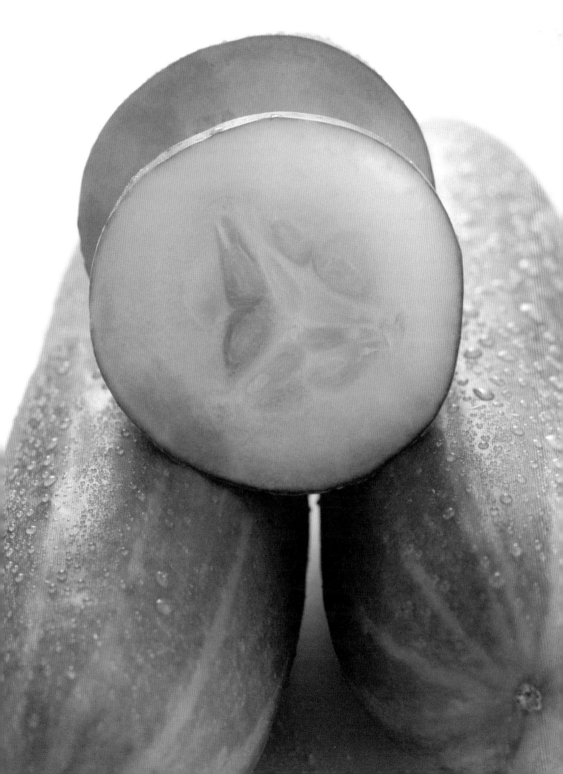

OUR RESEARCH RESULTS

Crackers are just carbohydrates, right? Wrong. Judging from the results of the survey, fats and saturates are an integral part of the average cheese biscuit. In fact, only three products – Rakusen's Matzo Crackers, Ryvita's High Fibre Crackerbread and Ryvita Original – contain less than 3g of fat per 100g. While it may come as no surprise that snack biscuits such as the Tuc Cheese Sandwich are high in fat (at 31.4g per 100g), some of the other products to get a red light include Orkney Original Oatcakes (23g) and Fox's Wholemeal Crackers (20.6g). Many other crackers, such as Nairn's Rough Oat Cakes and WeightWatchers Cracked Black Pepper Savoury Biscuits follow closely behind with an amber rating. In many cases this will be due to the use of oil (or in the case of McVitie's Butter Puffs, butter) as a binding ingredient.

The figures for saturates are equally alarming. 100g of Cheddars contain 16g of saturated fats – that's 4g higher than any product in the Crisps table. And they're not alone: Tuc Original, Tuc Cheese Sandwich, Jacob's Ritz Cheese Sandwich and McVitie's Butter Puffs all contain more than 14g saturated fat per 100g. They are also salty: Ritz Crackers come out highest with 3.3g per 100g, followed by Jacob's Hovis Wheatgerm Crackers, Jacob's Ritz Cheese Sandwich and Torinesi Breadsticks at 2.5g. The only product in the table to contain no added salt is Rakusen's Matzo Crackers. Lowest in calories are Ryvita Originals with 317kcal per 100g.

THE GOOD NUTRITION GUIDE RECOMMENDS

LOWEST IN SUGARS:
Orkney Original Oatcakes

LOWEST IN SATURATED FATS:
Rakusen's Matzo Crackers; Ryvita Original

LOWEST IN SALT:
Rakusen's Matzo Crackers

THE GOOD NUTRITION GUIDE BEST CHOICE:
Rakusen's Matzo Crackers

Brand Name	Energy	Protein	Fibre	Carbohydrates	Sugars	Fat	Saturated Fat	Salt	Good Nutrition Guide Score	Company group
Carr's Table Water Biscuits With Sesame Seeds	416.0	10.5	4.4	70.6	1.5	10.2	3.5	1.5	62.0	Carr's
Carr's Table Water Biscuits	406.0	10.1	4.2	74.2	1.6	7.6	3.3	1.5	62.0	Carr's
Ferro's Lightly Salted Breadsticks	467.0	12.5	3.6	64.3	3.5	17.8	7.1	2.0	37.5	Ferro's
Fox's Wholemeal Crackers	455.0	8.5	7.2	59.0	13.3	20.6	7.8	1.6	12.5	Fox's
Pagen Wholegrain Krisprolls	370.0	12.0	9.5	65.0	6.5	7.0	1.0	1.8	50.0	G.Costa & Co
Torinesi Breadsticks	413.0	9.9	4.0	69.5	3.5	10.5	5.0	2.5	50.0	Grissin Bon
Nairn's Rough Oat Cakes	429.0	10.4	7.6	57.1	0.7	17.7	3.5	1.2	62.5	Nairn's
Delser Italian Crackers	450.0	10.6	3.3	72.8	2.2	12.9	5.9	1.6	37.5	Quality Food Group
Rakusen's Matzo Crackers	369.0	10.5	3.6	82.9	1.4	1.1	0.3	0.0	100.0	Rakusen's
High Fibre Crackerbread	355.0	12.5	15.0	62.4	1.4	2.8	0.5	1.0	87.5	Ryvita
Ryvita Original	317.0	8.5	16.5	66.9	2.9	1.7	0.3	0.5	87.5	Ryvita
Simmers Macvita	447.0	8.7	11.3	61.6	10.3	13.3	5.9	2.0	25.0	Simmers of Edinburgh
Orkney Original Oatcakes	453.0	11.1	6.0	50.3	0.3	23.0	6.1	1.9	25.0	Stockan & Gardens
Cheddars	509.0	11.6	2.7	53.2	3.5	27.6	16.0	1.5	37.5	United Biscuits
Jacob's Choice Grain Crackers	427.0	9.0	5.4	65.5	5.2	14.3	6.4	1.8	25.0	United Biscuits
Jacob's Cream Cracker	431.0	10.0	3.8	67.6	1.4	13.5	6.2	1.3	50.0	United Biscuits
Jacob's Essentials Whole Wheat Crackers	381.0	14.8	7.9	62.3	1.6	8.1	1.1	0.5	75.0	United Biscuits
Jacob's Hovis Wheatgerm Crackers	447.0	10.2	4.4	60.0	6.8	18.5	9.7	2.5	25.0	United Biscuits
Jacob's Ritz Cheese Sandwich	527.0	9.4	2.1	56.2	6.9	29.3	20.3	2.5	12.5	United Biscuits
McVities Butter Puffs	493.0	8.3	3.1	57.7	1.2	25.5	14.1	1.0	37.5	United Biscuits
McVities Crackerwheat	446.0	9.7	5.8	60.0	2.7	18.6	9.4	1.8	37.5	United Biscuits
Ritz Crackers	493.0	7.0	5.9	57.5	6.6	26.1	12.3	3.3	12.5	United Biscuits
Tuc Cheese Sandwich	531.0	8.4	2.3	53.8	4.0	31.4	15.6	1.5	37.5	United Biscuits
Tuc Original	522.0	7.0	2.9	60.5	5.3	28.0	22.0	1.8	12.5	United Biscuits
Finn Crisp Wheat & Poppy Crisp Bread	390.0	10.0	5.8	72.0	4.7	6.7	1.0	1.3	75.0	Vassan & Vassan
Weight Watchers Cracked Black pepper Savoury Biscuits	446.0	8.3	9.4	59.2	2.8	19.5	5.2	0.6	50.0	Walkers Shortbread

Key

Typical serving size: 100g (quarter of a quiche)

All figures are grammes per 100 grammes (expect Energy reading which = Kcal per100 grammes)

Source: The Ethical Company Organisation / The Good Nutrition Guide 2006 - 2008

For explantion of Good Nutrition Guide Score see the "Using the Research Tables" section

The Good Nutrition Guide

Worst Choice:

Fox's Wholemeal Crackers; Jacob's Ritz
Cheese Sandwich; Ritz Crackers;
Tuc Original

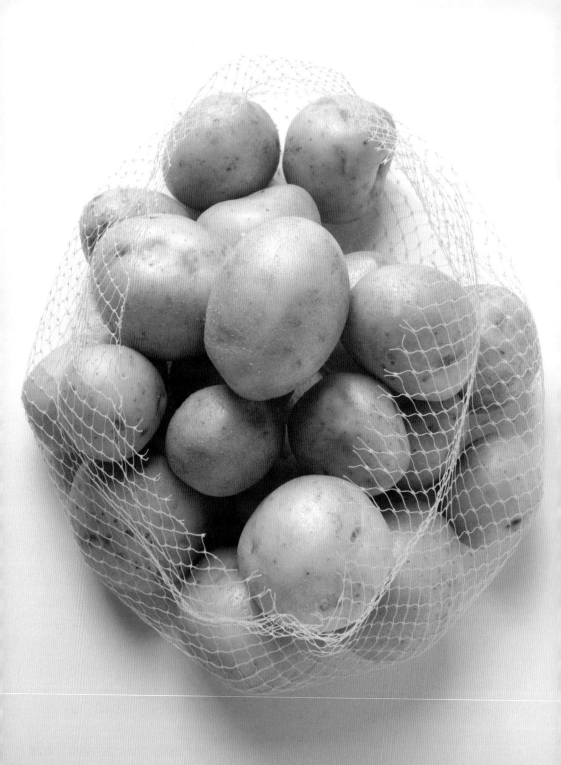

Chips and Potato Snacks

Whether served in a microwaveable carton or yesterday's newspaper, chips are the ultimate fast food: both a satisfying side dish and a meal in themselves. With the addition of wedges, waffles and curly fries to the chip roster, the potential choice of potato snacks is bigger than ever. While chips will never be a healthy substitute for good old baked spuds, there is no doubt that they are improving, and some (although far from all) brands can now boast significantly lower levels of salt and fat.

LOTS OF STARCHES

According to the British Potato Council, 2 million potatoes are made into chips in Britain each year – that's one in four of the potatoes harvested in the UK, and an awful lot of salt, vinegar and vegetable oil. Traditional chips are made from starchy potatoes, which are fried twice to remove most of the water. This is what makes them crispy on the outside and light on the inside.

Due to their high starch content, chips cause a huge temporary rise in blood sugar, which is why you often feel hungry again soon after eating them. On the glycaemic index, a scale that measures the effect of foods on blood glucose levels, they score a very high 95 out of 100. This means that they are digested quickly and release a burst of glucose into the body, but don't provide the slow-release energy of low-GI foods.

POLYUNSATURATED FATS

The nutritional value of a chip is partly dependent on the type of fat it is fried in. Polyunsaturated and monounsaturated fats are better for us than saturated fats, because they play a role in lowering (rather than raising) the levels of LDL cholesterol in our blood. Many manufacturers use sunflower oil, which is high in polyunsaturated fats. Corn and soya oils are also predominantly polyunsaturated, while olive and rapeseed oils consist mainly of monounsaturated fat.

While unsaturated fats are a better

option, they should still only be consumed in small quantities, particularly when they are a part of fried foods such as chips. Thick-cut or chunky chips are generally healthier than thinner fries because they absorb less oil. Nevertheless, as far as take-aways go, fish and chips are not the fattiest: according to the British Nutrition Foundation, the average portion of fish and chips contains almost three times less fat than a chicken tikka masala and rice.

TRAFFIC LIGHT LABELLING

Under the new signposting system for food packaging, one manufacturer – McCain – can display green circles for saturates, sugar and salt on the label for its Original Oven Chips. The chips also receive an amber circle for moderate levels of fat. This news has been greeted with ambivalence, as some groups have praised the company for reducing its salt and saturates levels, while others expressed concern that the traffic light labels could encourage consumers to believe that chips were a healthy option.

Even if they are low in fat, chips are not as nutritious as potatoes cooked in other ways. Jacket potatoes, for example, contain

no added fats or oils, and retain the nutrients found in the skin of the potato. The good nutrition advice is to use the traffic light labels to pick a product that is low in sugar, salt and saturates, but treat chips as an occasional treat regardless of their apparent credentials. Check whether the nutritional information is given for the frozen product, as the figures will usually increase when it is cooked.

OVEN CHIPS AND POTATO SNACKS

It's now relatively easy to find standard oven chips that contain nothing but potatoes and olive oil. Some companies have also removed the added salt from their products. Perhaps surprisingly, microwaveable chips are often as ingredient-light as the oven-ready options, although whether they taste as good is down to individual preference. However, as soon as you deviate away from oven chips into potato snacks – such as waffles, shapes and spicy chips – the additives return. All of these products are more likely to contain extra stabilisers, raising agents and starches, plus added sugars such as dextrose.

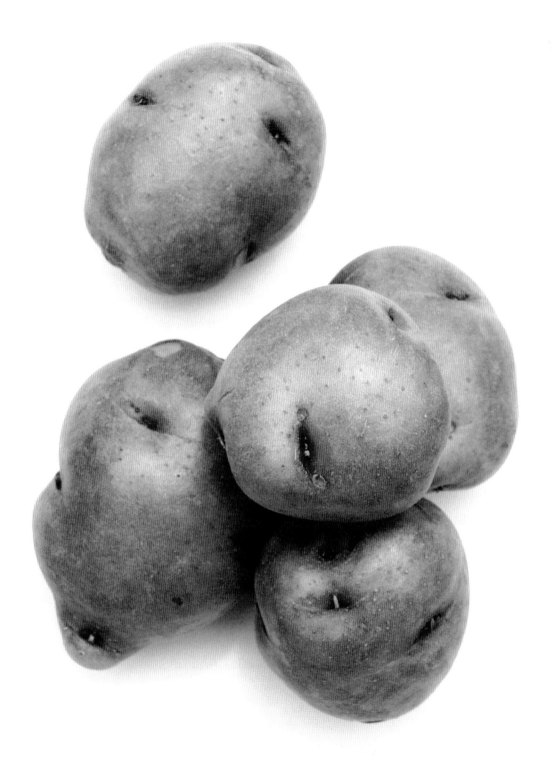

OUR RESEARCH RESULTS

A quick scan of the table might suggest that chips are healthier than expected. However, the figures given are for 100g of frozen product, so the numbers in some categories (particularly fat) are likely to increase once the food is cooked. Even so, two products in the table – McCain Oven Chips and McCain Micro Chips – receive three green lights for sugars, saturated fat and salt. All of the potato snacks surveyed have a low rating for sugars, with Aunt Bessie's Homestyle Chips displaying the highest figure at 1.0g per 100g. Aunt Bessies' is also the only other product to contain under 0.3g of salt per 100g.

Although the products are all rated amber for fat, there is still a big difference between the most and least fatty chips on offer. At the bottom of the list are Fries To Go with 12.8g fat per 100g, and at the top are McCain with just 4g. The rest fall somewhere in between, with McCain Hash Browns, McCain Rosti and Birds Eye Potato Waffles all displaying higher levels of fat. McCain's Hash Browns and Rosti are both amongst the highest in saturates, with 4.1g and 4.7g respectively, while Aunt Bessies' Homestyle Chips and Fries To Go also receive an amber

light. Of the remaining products, McCain Microchips are the lowest in saturates. They are also particularly low in salt.

While the table suggests that simple oven chips might be less unhealthy than potato snacks, it also shows that similar products are by no means equal. If in doubt, check the ingredients – the more potato in your chip, the better.

THE GOOD NUTRITION GUIDE RECOMMENDS

LOWEST IN SUGARS:
Birds Eye Potato Waffles

LOWEST IN SATURATED FATS:
Micro Chips

LOWEST IN SALT:
McCain Oven Chips; Micro Chips

THE GOOD NUTRITION GUIDE BEST CHOICE:
McCain Oven Chips; Micro Chips

THE GOOD NUTRITION GUIDE WORST CHOICE:
Fries To Go; McCain Hash Browns; McCain Rosti

BRAND NAME	ENERGY	PROTEIN	FIBRE	CARBOHYDRATES	SUGARS	FAT	SATURATED FAT	SALT	GOOD NUTRITION GUIDE SCORE	Company group
Aunt Bessie's Homestyle Chips	191	3.1	2.9	27	1.0	7.8	4.4	0.3	75.0	Aunt Bessie's
Fries To Go	305	3.7	3.4	43.9	0.5	12.8	2.5	0.6	62.5	Fries To Go
McCain Crispy French Fries	172	2.7	1.8	25.1	0.5	6.8	0.9	0.7	75.0	McCain
McCain Crispy Slices	163	2.1	1.4	21.9	0.6	5.7	0.6	0.4	75.0	McCain
McCain Hash Browns	164	1	2.8	19.9	0.5	9.0	4.1	0.8	62.5	McCain
McCain Homefries	134	2.2	1.7	21	0.5	4.6	0.6	0.5	75.0	McCain
McCain Oven Chips	138	2.5	1.9	26.2	0.6	4.0	0.6	0.2	87.5	McCain
McCain Potato Winners Wedges	144	2	1.7	20.8	0.6	5.9	0.6	0.6	75.0	McCain
McCain Rosti	169	2.2	1.8	19.6	0.8	9.1	4.7	0.7	62.5	McCain
McCain Smiles	191	2.6	2.7	27	0.5	8.0	1.0	0.7	75.0	McCain
Micro Chips	156	2.3	2	26.4	0.5	4.5	0.5	0.2	87.5	McCain
Birds Eye Potato Waffles	167	2	1.5	20.7	0.3	8.5	1.0	0.8	75.0	Birds Eye

Key

TYPICAL SERVING SIZE: 100G

All figures are grammes per 100 grammes (expect Energy reading which = Kcal per100 grammes)

Source: The Ethical Company Organisation / The Good Nutrition Guide 2006 - 2008

For explantion of Good Nutrition Guide Score see the "Using the Research Tables" section

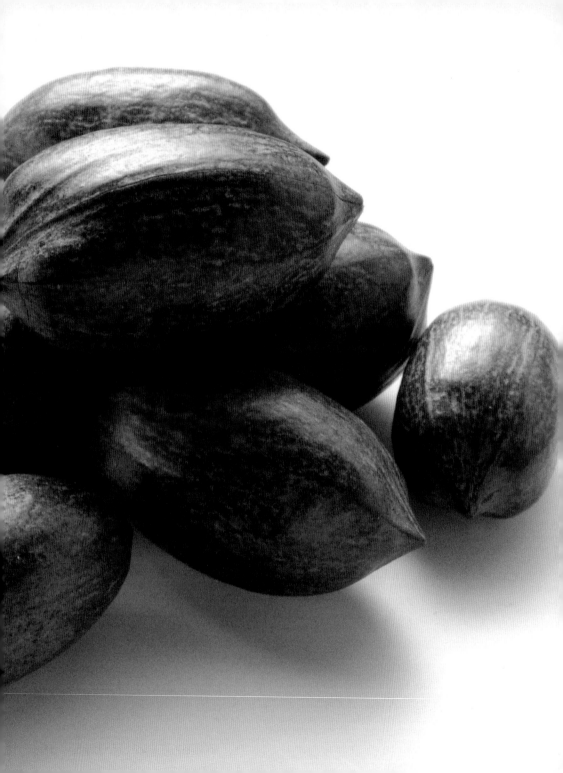

Chocolate

Every few months a new theory emerges about the nutritional benefits of chocolate, such as claims that it can help prevent heart disease, or protect you against cancer, or contains chemicals that mimic the feeling of being in love. The good news is that some of these stories might be more than just wishful thinking; the bad news is that any positive effects of eating chocolate will be tempered by the fact that it is full of both sugars and fats. Try dark chocolate, which is higher in cocoa solids and lower in sugar.

HISTORY OF CHOCOLATE

The Aztecs, who used the crushed seeds of the cacao tree in cooking and beverages, were the first people to recognise the potential of chocolate. Travellers bought the seeds back to Europe, where they were sweetened with sugar and made into a paste as the basis for chocolate drinks. By the late 1800s they had became part of the solid chocolate bars we know today.

The quality of a bar of chocolate is determined by the percentage of cocoa solids it contains. A good dark chocolate will be 60-75 per cent cocoa solids. It will usually contain some sugar, but retain the slight bitterness of unsweetened chocolate. Milk chocolates typically contain far lower percentages of cocoa solids – as little as 10

to 20 per cent in some cases. The addition of milk to cocoa solids gives the products their smoothness, but also contributes to chocolate's notoriously high fat content. White chocolate isn't technically chocolate, as it is produced from cocoa butter with added milk and sugar rather than cocoa beans. It is often the sweetest type of chocolate.

ADDED INGREDIENTS

The cocoa solids in chocolate bars are often labelled as "cocoa mass" in the ingredients; the nearer they come to the end of the list the less cocoa is in the product. In many milk and white chocolate bars, the main ingredient will be sugar, followed by milk. Most milk chocolates use either milk powder or dried cream in their recipes.

Chocolate bars often contain added fats such as palm or coconut oil or vegetable fat. These aren't good for the heart, so a better option is to pick chocolates that just include cocoa butter. There are some suggestions that the saturated fats from stearic and oleic acids in chocolate may have a more limited effect on the levels of LDL (bad) cholesterol in the blood than saturates from other sources. Nevertheless, chocolate still contains a high overall level of fat – and watch out for hydrogenated oils, which may indicate that trans fats are present.

The purest chocolates will contain just cocoa mass, cocoa butter and sugar, plus an emulsifier such as soya lecithin. If you are concerned about genetically modified foodstuffs, check that the soya hasn't come from a GM source. Many bars also include artificial flavourings and colourings, which will be named in the ingredients list.

Chocolate naturally contains caffeine. There are about 10g of caffeine in a standard chocolate bar – not enough to have a significant effect, unless you are also drinking lots of strong coffee (at 150mg per cup) or tea (at 50mg per cup). White chocolate tends to be lowest in caffeine.

NUTRITIONAL BENEFITS

When women claim to crave chocolate, they may actually be responding to a genuine nutritional need – good quality chocolate is high in magnesium, which the body seems to require in greater quantities at certain times during the menstrual cycle. Some studies have suggested that magnesium deficiency is a contributory cause of PMT, so the occasional indulgence might even be justifiable on health grounds!

Cocoa also contains antioxidants, which are the agents that appear in red wine and green tea and are thought to help protect against cancer and heart disease. These are found in much higher proportions in chocolates with lots of cocoa solids, which suggests that dark chocolate may be better for you than the milk and white varieties.

OUR RESEARCH RESULTS

It probably goes without saying that the Chocolate table is awash with low marks for sugars, fats and saturates, but amongst the sea of red are some good indicators

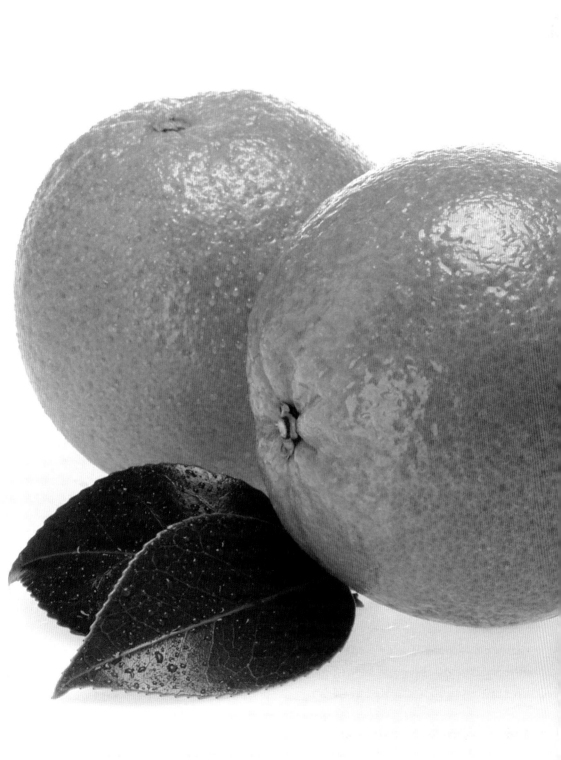

as to the quality of chocolate on offer. Of particular interest is the amount of sugar per 100g, which shows whether the chocolate has been highly sweetened or retains some of the bitterness of cocoa. Lindt Excellence is the only product in the table to get an amber light for sugar. At 15g per 100g, it has over a quarter of the sugar contained in Masterfoods' Milky Way bar, which has a staggering 66.6g per 100g. Lower sugar chocolates include Thorntons Dark Chocolate Gingers and Green & Black's Organic Dark 70%.

The disadvantage to this low sugar count is that it is usually accompanied by an increase in fat. Green & Black's Organic Dark 70% follows this rule with 41.1g per 100g, as does Lindt Excellence at 46g. However, in these cases the high fat content is likely to be due to extra cocoa butter rather than added oils – check the ingredients list to be sure. Lowest in saturates is the Milky Way, with 9.8g per 100g and the Mars bar, at 9.9g. Maltesers – marketed as a "lighter" chocolate product – contain 14.5g per 100g.

Despite all the sugar, there is also a significant amount of salt in some of these chocolates – only three products (Cadbury Bournville, Green & Black's Organic Dark

70% and Thorntons Dark Chocolate Gingers) contain a trace or less. With 0.8g, a Cadbury Crunchie contains the same amount of salt per 100g as Birds Eye Potato Waffles.

THE GOOD NUTRITION GUIDE RECOMMENDS

LOWEST IN SUGARS:
Lindt Excellence

LOWEST IN SATURATED FATS:
Milky Way

LOWEST IN SALT:
Bournville; Green & Black's Organic Dark 70%; Thorntons Dark Chocolate Gingers

THE GOOD NUTRITION GUIDE BEST CHOICE:
Lindt Excellence; Thorntons Dark Chocolate Gingers

THE GOOD NUTRITION GUIDE WORST CHOICE:
Dairy Milk Caramel; Snickers; Twix; Toffee Crisp

Brand Name	Energy	Protein	Fibre	Carbohydrates	Sugars	Fat	Saturated Fat	Salt	Good Nutrition Guide Score	Company group
Bournville	495	4	6	61.1	59.9	26.3	16.3	0.0	25.0	Cadbury Schweppes
Crunchie	470	4	0.5	71.8	57.0	18.3	10.8	0.8	25.0	Cadbury Schweppes
Diary Milk	525	7.7	0.7	56.9	56.5	29.7	18.3	0.3	25.0	Cadbury Schweppes
Dairy Milk Caramel	495	5.6	0.5	60.8	52.3	25.2	14.9	0.5	12.5	Cadbury Schweppes
Dairy Milk Fruit & Nut	490	8	1.4	55.5	55.0	26.4	14.0	0.3	25.0	Cadbury Schweppes
Green & Black's Organic Dark 70%	551	9.3	11.5	36	29.4	41.1	24.2	0.0	25.0	Cadbury Schweppes
Green & Black's Organic White	573	7.4	0.1	53.5	50.8	36.6	22.3	0.2	25.0	Cadbury Schweppes
Snaps	505	6.3	1	60.5	52.5	27.0	15.6	0.3	25.0	Cadbury Schweppes
Twirl Twin Bars	530	7.5	0.8	56.1	55.7	30.8	19.0	0.3	25.0	Kraft
Toblerone	530	5.4	2.6	58	57.0	30.5	18.0	0.1	37.0	Lindt & Sprungli
Lindt Excellence	520	11	0	19	15.0	46.0	27.0	0.1	25.0	Lir Chocolates
Baileys Truffles	506	5.2	1.3	57.6	52.5	28.9	17.6	0.2	25.0	Masterfoods
Bounty	469	3.7	2.2	63.8	47.8	23.9	19.8	0.3	25.0	Masterfoods
Galaxy	543	6.8	1.5	57.6	56.4	31.6	18.7	0.3	25.0	Masterfoods
Maltesers	505	7.9	1.1	62.8	53.8	24.7	14.5	0.2	25.0	Masterfoods
Mars	455	4.1	1.3	69.7	59.5	17.7	9.9	0.5	25.0	Masterfoods
Mars Delight	557	4.5	1.4	58.9	44.5	33.6	21.3	0.2	25.0	Masterfoods
Milky Way	454	3.5	0.6	72	66.6	16.9	9.8	0.6	25.0	Masterfoods
Ripple	531	6.7	1.4	60.3	58.9	29.3	16.9	0.2	12.5	Masterfoods
Snickers	501	9.3	2.5	52.9	45.4	28.1	11.1	0.6	12.5	Masterfoods
Twix	492	4.7	1.5	65.1	49.3	23.7	13.5	0.4	25.0	Nestle
Aero	533	4.9	0.4	61.2	61.0	29.8	18.9	0.2	25.0	Nestle
KitKat Chunky	518	5.2	1	60.9	50.8	28.2	19.3	0.2	25.0	Nestle
Nestle Milkybar	543	7.6	0	57.6	57.6	31.3	20.3	0.3	12.5	Nestle
Toffee Crisp	516	3.8	1	63.1	48.9	27.6	12.6	0.5	25.0	Nestle
Thorntons Brazil Nuts	588	17.2	3.2	36.9	36.1	44.3	18.8	0.1	25.0	Thorntons
Thorntons Dark Chocolate Gingers	259	4.2	4.8	23.5	17.6	16.6	10.2	0.0	37.5	Thorntons

Key

Typical serving size: 40g (one bar)

All figures are grammes per 100 grammes (expect Energy reading which = Kcal per 100 grammes)

Source: The Ethical Company Organisation / The Good Nutrition Guide 2006 - 2008

For explantion of Good Nutrition Guide Score see the "Using the Research Tables" section

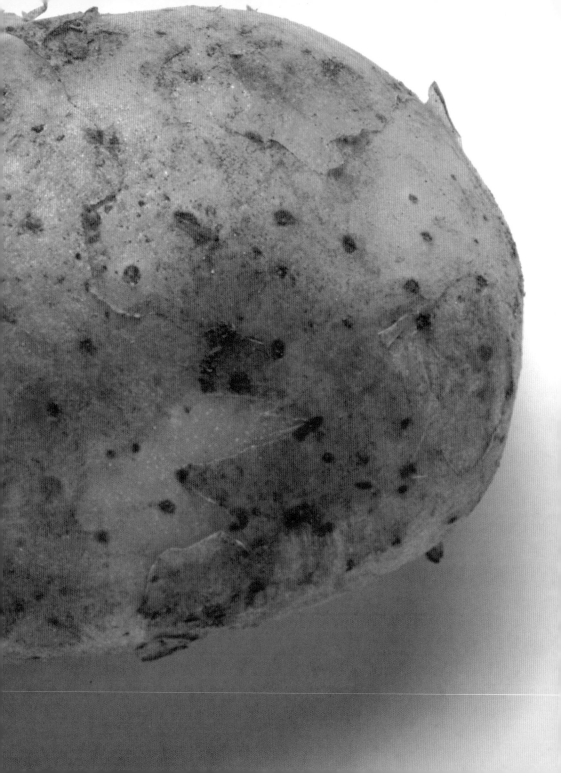

Crisps

According to the Food Standards Agency, 9 billion packets of crisps and nuts, or the equivalent of 150 bags per person, are eaten every year in the UK. Three bags of crisps a week may not sound like much, but in terms of nutritional value it's a lot of empty calories. And a lot of wasted money: by cutting out most of your 150 bags you could save around £50 a year. Naturally, the snack industry would like you to continue parting with your cash, but are its efforts to redefine the crisp, and its fat content, enough for the health-conscious consumer?

"What Goes Into Crisps Goes Into You"

In response to concerns about the effects of saturated fat on cardiac health, the British Heart Foundation launched a poster campaign in September 2006 based upon its calculation that children who eat a packet of crisps every day are taking in almost five litres of cooking oil per year. The image of a girl drinking from a bottle of oil was criticised for using scare tactics, but it brought the BHF's underlying message – that "what goes into crisps goes into you" – into the spotlight.

The BHF found that a standard 35g bag of crisps contains two and a half teaspoons of oil. According to its research, one in five children aged 8-15 eats two packets of crisps per day, meaning that they could be consuming over nine litres of cooking oil a year. Although crisps are a particularly popular addition to school lunchboxes, it is not just children who should be heeding the BHF's warning – even as adults we are a nation of crisp lovers, responsible for half the total crisp sales in the EU.

A Healthy Crisp?

Crisp manufacturers have already started responding to criticisms that their products contribute to unhealthy diets and are helping to fuel the problem of obesity. Walkers were amongst the first to change their recipe, reducing levels of salt and saturated fat in a number of their ranges.

They have done this by frying the crisps in oil made from sunflower seeds, which contains higher levels of monounsaturates and lower levels of saturates than traditional oils. The standard Walkers bag now contains a maximum of 0.9g of saturated fat, which is 70 per cent lower than in 2003.

While dieticians have broadly welcomed this move, there are concerns that rebranding crisps as "healthy" may cause further confusion amongst consumers. Even after any reductions in saturated fat have been taken into account, they are still a high-fat, high calorie snack. Also, the reductions Walkers have made do not apply to every brand in their range – a fact that has already led the company to fall foul of the Advertising Standards Authority for misrepresenting the extent of the changes. Nevertheless, it is only a matter of time before the low-salt, low-saturates message filters through to the rest of the snack industry.

How Many Crisps in a Bag?

Research has found that people tend to eat whatever size of portion they are given, so someone who buys a bag of crisps offering "50 per cent extra free" is unlikely to save the "free" crisps for later. Our idea of a portion of crisps is constantly being modified by the trend for bigger versions of familiar products.

Although a standard packet of crisps usually weighs in at 35g, many companies now offer an extra-large bag of 50g or more. Multipack bags tend to be smaller at 25g, so by choosing to buy more crisps you may actually be eating less per portion. This option is certainly better than the "family" or "share" size packs, where an individual serving is much more difficult to define – unless you happen to have access to some weighing scales.

Vegetables and Other Alternatives

Vegetable crisps, particularly those made from parsnip and beetroot, have rapidly increased in popularity in recent years. While they might seem preferable to ordinary potato crisps, it is important to remember that any vitamins found in the original vegetables are likely to have been destroyed during the frying process. Where the vegetable variations do improve on standard crisps is that many

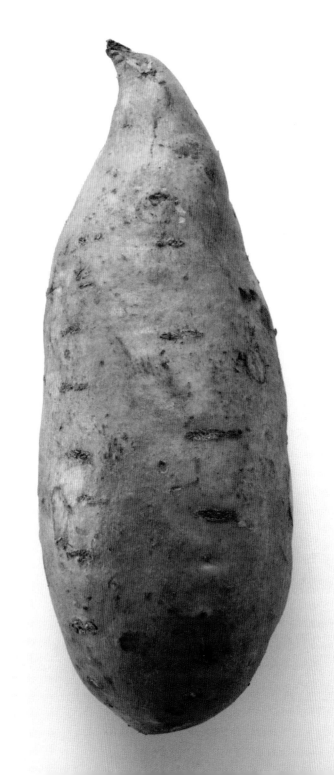

brands contain no added salt.

Thicker cut potato crisps – including more upmarket lines such as Kettle chips – may contain lower levels of oil than the thinnest varieties. Look for crisps that use unpeeled potatoes, as these will have a higher fibre content. Crisps based on corn rather than potatoes are unlikely to be healthier in terms of salt and fat, and as these brands tend to be aimed at children they often contain higher levels of flavourings and colours.

OUR RESEARCH RESULTS

Walkers have been criticised for not making it clear enough to consumers that their low fat drive does not extend to all products, and it is clear from the table that the Sensations range is not included – these products contain 9g of saturated fat per 100g as compared to 2.6g for the standard range. Interestingly, the figures for Kettle Chips show that they have similarly low saturates levels, plus lower levels of fat overall. The Pringles and Doritos ranges are both high in saturates, with many products containing 10g or more per 100g. The lowest overall fat figure in the table, 12.5g, is held by Jacob's

Original Twiglets.

Of the other nutrients, Walkers Wotsits are highest in sugar at 8.0g per 100g, and Walkers Oven Roasted Chicken With Lemon & Thyme are highest in salt with 3.6g per 100g. Lowest in salt are Doritos Lightly Salted Corn Chips at 0.8g per 100g. Jacob's Original Twiglets are by far the lowest in calories at 388kcal per 100g.

THE GOOD NUTRITION GUIDE RECOMMENDS

LOWEST IN SUGARS:
Hula Hoops

LOWEST IN SATURATED FATS:
Walkers Cheese & Onion; Walkers Prawn Cocktail; Walkers Ready Salted; Walkers Salt & Vinegar

LOWEST IN SALT:
Doritos Lightly Salted Corn Chips

THE GOOD NUTRITION GUIDE BEST CHOICE:
Kettle Chips Lightly Salted; Kettle Chips Salsa With Mesquite; Walkers Cheese & Onion

BRAND NAME	ENERGY	PROTEIN	FIBRE	CARBOHYDRATES	SUGARS	FAT	SATURATED FAT	SALT	GOOD NUTRITION GUIDE SCORE	Company group
KETTLE CHIPS LIGHTLY SALTED	482.0	6.3	5.1	56.0	0.9	25.8	2.9	0.9	50.0	Kettle Foods
KETTLE CHIPS MATURE CHEDDAR & CHIVE	478.0	8.1	5.0	54.4	3.6	25.4	3.3	1.7	37.5	Kettle Foods
KETTLE CHIPS SALSA WITH MESQUITE	469.0	6.0	5.2	56.4	3.9	24.4	2.7	1.4	50.0	Kettle Foods
KETTLE CHIPS SEA SALT & CRUSHED BLACK PEPPERCORNS	471.0	6.2	4.9	57.0	1.2	24.3	2.7	1.5	50.0	Kettle Foods
HULA HOOPS	514.0	3.2	1.8	61.5	0.4	28.4	6.1	2.5	25.0	KP Snacks
PRINGLES GOURMET FLAME-GRILLED STEAK & CARAMELISED ONION	511.0	4.7	3.6	52.0	3.9	30.0	11.0	2.1	25.0	Procter & Gamble
PRINGLES ORIGINAL	540.0	4.1	3.6	49.0	1.9	36.0	10.0	1.3	37.5	Procter & Gamble
PRINGLES SALT & VINEGAR	527.0	3.9	3.4	50.0	5.0	34.0	10.0	2.1	25.0	Procter & Gamble
PRINGLES SOUR CREAM & ONION	531.0	4.5	3.6	49.0	2.7	35.0	10.0	1.7	25.0	Procter & Gamble
PRINGLES THE CLASSIC ORIGINAL DIPPERS	524.0	5.0	3.9	53.0	2.1	32.0	11.0	1.4	37.5	Procter & Gamble
JACOB'S ORIGINAL TWIGLETS	388.0	12.8	11.8	56.1	2.1	12.5	5.5	1.8	37.5	United Biscuits
McVITIE'S BAKED MINI CHEDDARS	517.0	10.9	2.5	50.8	4.6	30.0	11.9	2.5	25.0	United Biscuits
DORITOS COOL ORIGINAL FLAVOUR CORN CHIPS	505.0	7.5	3.0	58.0	4.0	27.0	12.0	2.0	25.0	Walkers
DORITOS HINT OF LIME CORN CHIPS	500.0	6.5	3.0	60.0	1.9	26.0	12.0	1.3	37.5	Walkers
DORITOS LIGHTLY SALTED CORN CHIPS	495.0	7.0	3.0	63.0	1.0	24.0	11.0	0.8	37.5	Walkers
DORITOS TANGY CHEESE FLAVOUR CORN CHIPS	500.0	7.0	3.0	57.0	3.0	27.0	12.0	1.8	25.0	Walkers
SENSATIONS SLOW ROASTED LAMB WITH MOROCCAN SPICES	495.0	6.0	4.5	53.0	1.8	29.0	9.0	3.3	25.0	Walkers
WALKERS CHEESE & ONION	525.0	7.0	4.0	50.0	2.5	33.0	2.6	1.3	50.0	Walkers
WALKERS OVEN ROASTED CHICKEN WITH LEMON & THYME	500.0	6.5	4.0	53.0	3.0	29.0	9.0	3.6	25.0	Walkers
WALKERS PRAWN COCKTAIL	525.0	6.5	4.0	50.0	1.9	33.0	2.6	1.5	50.0	Walkers
WALKERS READY SALTED	530.0	6.5	4.0	49.0	0.5	34.0	2.6	1.5	50.0	Walkers
WALKERS SALT & VINEGAR	525.0	6.5	4.0	50.0	0.5	33.0	2.6	2.3	37.5	Walkers
WALKERS SENSATIONS THAI SWEET CHILLI	505.0	6.5	4.5	54.0	3.0	29.0	9.0	3.0	25.0	Walkers
WOTSITS	540.0	5.5	1.1	55.0	8.0	33.0	3.8	2.3	25.0	Walkers

Key

TYPICAL SERVING SIZE: 35G (one bag)

All figures are grammes per 100 grammes (expect Energy reading which = Kcal per100 grammes)

Source: The Ethical Company Organisation / The Good Nutrition Guide 2006 - 2008

For explantion of Good Nutrition Guide Score see the "Using the Research Tables" section

THE GOOD NUTRITION GUIDE
WORST CHOICE:

Hula Hoops; Pringles Gourmet Flame-Grilled Steak & Caramelised Onion; Pringles Salt & Vinegar; Pringles Sour Cream & Onion; McVitie's Baked Mini Cheddars; Doritos Cool Original Flavour Corn Chips; Doritos Tangy Cheese Flavour Corn Chips; Sensations Slow Roasted Lamb With Moroccan Spices; Walkers Oven Roasted Chicken With Lemon & Thyme; Walkers Sensations Thai Sweet Chilli; Wotsits

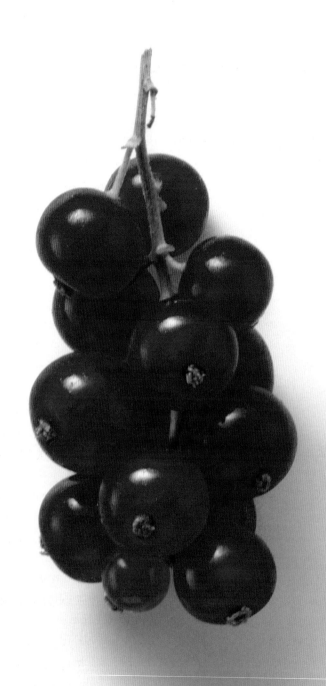

Frozen Desserts

Rows upon rows of mouth-watering sponge puddings, scrumptious cheesecakes and gluttonous gateaux: the freezer cabinet is where the best of intentions are destroyed. All of these tempting treats are packed with fats and sugars, and the prospect of a low-calorie version – well, that defies the point, really, doesn't it? As with most of the unhealthiest treats, our cravings for indulgence might be best served with an occasional, good-quality dessert made from natural ingredients, rather than regular consumption of the additive-filled "diet" alternatives.

A Sweet Tooth

All frozen desserts are high in fat and sugar, but the levels of these nutrients vary widely according to the type of pudding. Cheesecakes are particularly high in fat because they contain large quantities of cream and cream cheese. Pavlovas and roulades – which are based on meringue – are mostly sugar, but may also be fatty if they are filled with cream. Gateaux and sponge cakes are likely to fall in between the two, depending on the type of icing and filling used. For a general guide, the Food Standards Agency considers anything over 20g fat per 100g, or over 10g sugars per 100g, to be "a lot".

Fruit pies may have the theoretical advantage of added fibre and vitamin C, but check the ingredients to see if the fruit has been cooked in sugar or syrup. This may be listed as glucose, corn syrup or honey (amongst other terms) on the label. The pastry will probably be made from high-fat butter, which is a source of saturates and may also contain trans fats if hydrogenated vegetable oil is present. Choose open-topped or deep-filled pies, as these will have proportionally more fruit to pastry.

Reduced Fat and Sugar

Supermarket freezer cabinets are full of puddings proclaiming themselves "reduced fat" or diet-friendly, but although these products may be a good option if you are looking to reduce your calorie intake, they aren't necessarily more nutritious than the standard equivalent. Diet foods often require more processing to produce the same taste and texture with less of the key ingredients, which usually means that the product will contain extra additives.

Reducing a product's fat content may involve substituting regular ingredients for less fatty versions – such as skimmed milk instead of whole – or just using less of the ingredient overall. Low sugar foods usually contain artificial sweeteners, many of which are calorie-free, and flavourings may be used to mimic the richness of the original product. However, frozen foods often use fewer preservatives in comparison to refrigerated ones, so if you are concerned about added ingredients they are often a good choice.

Given that desserts are by their nature unhealthy, the key to finding the most nutritional choice may be buying the product with the best quality ingredients and the fewest additives. Perhaps contrarily, finding the "healthy option" may mean picking the full fat, full sugar dessert – and simply eating less of it.

OPTIONAL EXTRAS

Most desserts wouldn't be complete without extras such as cream, ice cream or crème fraîche. Go for lower fat options, such as single instead of double cream. While double cream can contain more than 50 per cent fat, single cream contains about 20 per cent – a significant reduction if you are looking to lessen your fat intake. It is also possible to buy dairy-free soya cream, which does still contain fat (usually in the form of vegetable oil) but also has the nutritional benefits of soya. Better still, use natural yoghurt, fromage frais or fresh fruit such as strawberries. Frozen yoghurt may be a good alternative to ice cream.

Once a product has been defrosted it usually has to be eaten within one day. If you know you won't need an entire pudding, it may be possible to defrost just half of the dessert – removing the incentive to scoff the rest inside 24 hours! It may also be helpful to compare the frozen dessert with an equivalent single-serving option from the chiller cabinet.

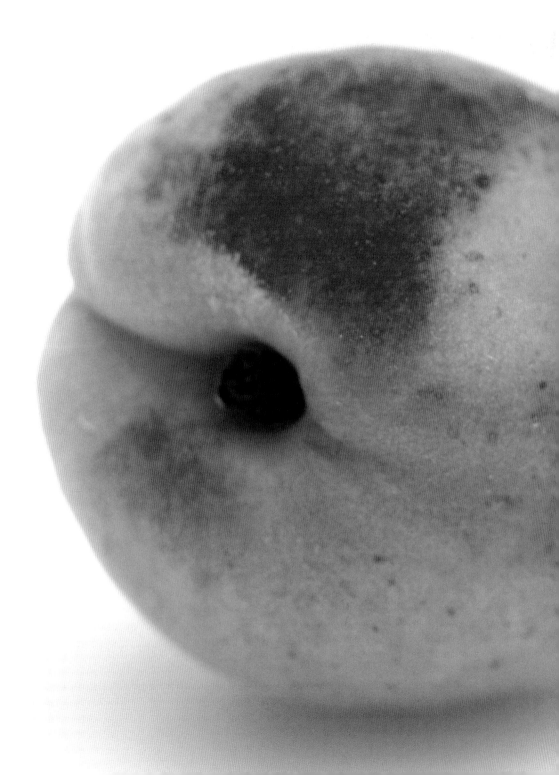

OUR RESEARCH RESULTS

The main concerns for frozen desserts are fats and sugars, and all of the products surveyed have these aplenty. Highest for fats are Aunt Bessie's Ready To Bake Chocolate Chip Cookies with a huge 23.8g of fat per 100g – a full 5g more than its nearest rival, the Devonshire Classics Lemon Pie. Both of these puddings also contain large quantities of saturates, with double the amount classified as "high" by the Food Standards Agency. In contrast, the two Scooby Doo Puds in the table have less than 1.5g of saturates per 100g. With low values for fats and sugars, these come out best overall – a good result for a product targeted at children. Perhaps surprisingly, Countrystyle Foods' Real Dairy Cream Doughnuts are much lower in sugar than many of the other products, although they make up for this with a lot of fat and saturates.

For each of the categories there is a great deal of variation between products, suggesting that even amongst "treat" foods there is still space for differing nutritional choices. For example, the Aunt Bessie's brand scored less well for salt, with two desserts (Ready To Bake Bramley Apple Crumble and Ready To Bake Lemon Meringue Pie) receiving a red light at 1.8g per 100g. The rest of the desserts, in comparison, had salt levels of 0.5g per 100g or less. The ranges for fats and saturates were similarly diverse, although the table brought good news for buyers of slimming products: the WeightWatchers Cookies 'n' Cream Sundae was by far the lowest in calories.

THE GOOD NUTRITION GUIDE RECOMMENDS

LOWEST IN SUGARS:
Scooby Doo Jam Sponge & Custard Paw Puds

LOWEST IN SATURATED FATS:
Scooby Doo Chocolate Sponge Paw Puds

LOWEST IN SALT:
WeightWatchers Cookies 'n' Cream Sundae

THE GOOD NUTRITION GUIDE BEST CHOICE:
Scooby Doo Chocolate Sponge Paw Puds; Scooby Doo Jam Sponge & Custard Paw Puds

BRAND NAME	ENERGY	PROTEIN	FIBRE	CARBOHYDRATES	SUGARS	FAT	SATURATED FAT	SALT	GOOD NUTRITION GUIDE SCORE	Company group
AMERICAN STYLE ALABAMA FUDGE CAKE	337	4.5	2.3	55.1	27.4	11.0	2.8	0.3	50.0	Bonne Bouche Frozen
SCOOBY DOO CHOCOLATE SPONGE PAW PUDS	214	4.5	2.1	34.2	14.0	6.5	1.0	0.5	62.5	Bonne Bouche Frozen
SCOOBY DOO JAM SPONGE & CUSTARD PAW PUDS	258	3.4	0.4	41	13.1	8.9	1.4	0.4	62.5	Bonne Bouche Frozen
REAL DAIRY CREAM DOUGHNUTS	315	5.9	1.6	43.3	14.0	13.8	7.9	0.5	37.5	Countrystyle Foods
DEVONSHIRE CLASSICS LEMON PIE	333	4.1	8.7	37.7	32.8	18.4	10.2	0.4	25.0	Heniz
DEVONSHIRE CLASSICS STRAWBERRY CHEESECAKE	242	4.1	2.9	28.3	20.9	12.5	6.9	0.3	37.5	Heniz
WEIGHTWATCHERS COOKIES 'N' CREAM SUNDAE	156	2.5	2.2	30.3	19.1	3.4	2.2	0.2	50.0	Heniz
ROSS STRAWBERRY CHEESECAKE	282	3.7	1.5	38.7	22.8	12.5	4.5	0.3	50.0	Ross Desserts
AUNT BESSIE'S READY TO BAKE BRAMLEY APPLE CRUMBLE	220	2.3	2.5	36.6	18.7	7.1	3.2	1.8	25.0	Tryton Foods
AUNT BESSIE'S READY TO BAKE LEMON MERINGUE PIE	288	3.8	2	49.8	30.4	8.2	2.7	1.8	25.0	Tryton Foods
AUNT BESSIE'S READY TO BAKE CHOCOLATE CHIP COOKIES	488	4.7	2.8	63.7	41.1	23.8	12.7	0.5	12.5	Tryton Foods

Key

TYPICAL SERVING SIZE: 100G

All figures are grammes per 100 grammes (expect Energy reading which = Kcal per100 grammes)

Source: The Ethical Company Organisation / The Good Nutrition Guide 2006 - 2008

For explantion of Good Nutrition Guide Score see the "Using the Research Tables" section

THE GOOD NUTRITION GUIDE
WORST CHOICE:
Aunt Bessie's Ready To Bake Chocolate
Chip Cookies

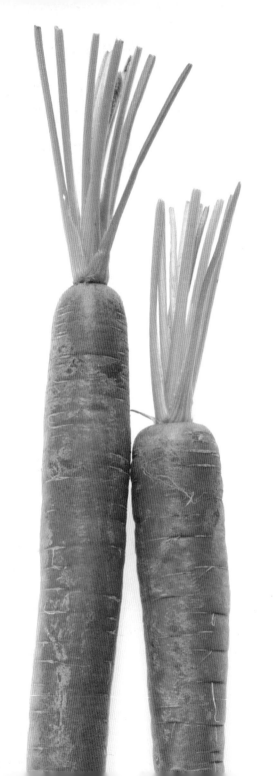

Gravy, Stock and Stuffing

It's the little things that make all the difference. Gravy granules, stock cubes and stuffing mixes are just some of the simple but effective products that make producing an otherwise time-consuming meal that much easier. But the necessary trade-off for this convenience, as ever, seems to be nutritional value. High in additives and flavourings, and low in meat and vegetables, many of these goods contain little of the protein or fibre found in home-cooked stocks and gravies – and are often a major source of hidden salt.

As Good as Home-Made?

Gravies, stocks and stuffing mixes are ideal labour-saving inventions. No longer does gravy have to be made from the fat of a slow-cooked roast, or stock boiled for hours before it is ready to use. These new products put the finishing touches to a meal in the time it takes to boil a kettle. However, in terms of nutritional value these items are often less impressive. A home-made stock may take time to cook, but it is guaranteed to contain fresh ingredients: meat, vegetables and herbs. The processed version may be a little lighter on the crucial components; how else could a "traditional" gravy be suitable for vegetarians?

In many cases, one of the main ingredients will be potato starch, which provides the product with its bulk. Dextrins – such as maltodextrin – are used as thickeners. Most stocks and gravies contain a few dried herbs or vegetable extracts, but rely on flavourings and flavour enhancers to fill the gaps. These often include monosodium glutamate, which is a further source of sodium and is often used to give crisps and other savoury foods their "moreish" quality.

While many manufacturers of high fat products such as margarines and cakes are removing hydrogenated vegetable oils from their products due to concern about trans fats, these oils are still relatively common (albeit in very small quantities) in gravies and stocks. They may also appear in stuffing mixes. Look for mixes that use wholemeal bread, as this contains more fibre and other nutrients than white, and try products that include fresh or dried herbs rather than flavourings.

HIGH SALT FOODS

Gravies and stocks often contain more than 0.5g of sodium per 100g of the finished product, which means that they are high in salt. Oxo's Vegetable Stock Cubes, for example, list salt as the main ingredient – meaning that each cube was made with more salt by weight than anything else. If this is surprising then it could be that you (like much of the population) are consuming too much "hidden" salt in your diet.

The nutrition label often gives two sets of figures, one for 100g dry weight and one per serving. As the products are usually heavily diluted at home, the per serving figure may be more helpful. Choose low salt options where possible, and if the food is too dry top it up with water rather than extra stock. Avoid seasoning the meal until after the gravy or stock has been added, as these may provide more than enough salt in themselves.

OTHER ISSUES

During the BSE crisis, some stock manufacturers removed the beef from their products to allay public fears that the disease may be spread to humans through the food chain. The most prominent company to change its recipe was Bovril, which began making its beef-extract spreads and stocks with a vegetarian yeast extract. This decision has been reversed since the EU lifted its export ban on British beef, but non-meat gravies and stocks have nevertheless become more widely available in recent years.

There have also been other expansions in the gravy/stock market, particularly into products that offer blends of herbs and spices based on Italian, Indian and Chinese cuisine. Like the more conventional stock cubes, these are frequently high in salt and packed with additives. For a true taste of other cultures it would be more authentic – and, in the long run, cheaper – to buy the individual spices. The same is true of granulated sauces, which rarely replicate the nutritional content of a home-made equivalent.

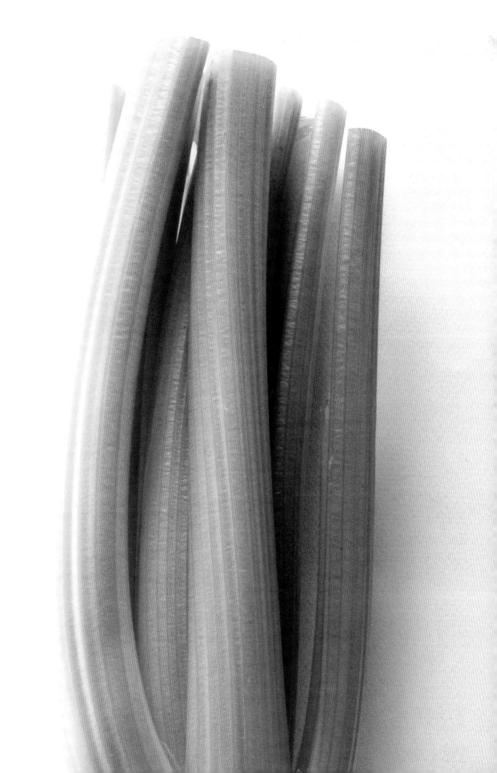

Our Research Results

Stock and stock cubes are notoriously high in salt: Knorr Chicken Stock Granules and Marigold Swiss Vegetable Bouillon Powder both contain a massive 44g per 100g. While the good news is that these stocks are only used in small, diluted quantities, the bad news is that salt may still be a factor; the recommended serving of 5g of Marigold Bouillon dissolved in 250ml water contains 2.25g of salt. Nevertheless, this works out at a similar figure per 100g to ready-made stocks such as Just Bouillon and Knorr Simply Stock.

Gravies can be equally salty – perhaps more so, given that they tend to be less heavily diluted than stocks. Bisto Favourite Gravy Granules and Oxo Gravy Granules For Roast Chicken contain 15.2g and 16g salt per 100g respectively. The Bisto product is significantly higher in fat, listing 9g of saturates per 100g to Oxo's 0.9g. Just Bouillon Red Meat Gravy and Schwartz Rich Onion Gravy are both even lower in fats, with Schwartz on just 0.2g fat per 100g.

The stuffing products surveyed are mostly low in fat; only Merchant Gourmet and Paxo Celebrations get an amber rating

in this category. Highest in sugars and calories is Sierra Rica Organic with 12.4g.

The Good Nutrition Guide Recommends

Lowest in Sugars:
Knorr Simply Stock Chicken; Knorr The Fish Cube

Lowest in Saturated fats:
Knorr Simply Stock Chicken

Lowest in Salt:
Sierra Rica Organic Traditional Chestnut Stuffing

the Good Nutrition Guide Best Choice:
Paxo Sage & Onion Stuffing; Chiltern Herbs Country Stuffing; Just Bouillon Chicken Stock; Just Bouillon Red Meat Gravy; Just Bouillon Concentrated Stock Vegetable; Schwartz Rich Onion Gravy; Shropshire Spice Co. Sage & Onion Stuffing Mix; Knorr Simply Stock Chicken; Knorr The Fish Cube

GRAVY, STOCK AND STUFFING MIX

BRAND NAME	ENERGY	PROTEIN	FIBRE	CARBOHYDRATES	SUGARS	FAT	SATURATED FAT	SALT	GOOD NUTRITION GUIDE SCORE	Company group
BISTO FAVOURITE GRAVY GRANULES	385	2.5	1.3	7.3	13.8	16.2	9.1	15.2	25.0	Premier Foods
PAXO CELEBRATIONS SAUSAGEMEAT & THYME	155	5.8	3	25.1	1.6	3.5	1.2	1.7	62.5	Premier Foods
PAXO SAGE & ONION STUFFING	143	3.2	1.9	29.9	0.9	1.2	0.5	0.9	87.5	Premier Foods
OXO BEEF	265	17.3	1.5	38.4	2.6	4.7	2.3	27.3	50.0	Campbell Grocery Products
OXO GRAVY GRANULES FOR ROAST CHICKEN	311	10.2	0.7	63.1	7.4	2.0	0.9	16.0	62.5	Campbell Grocery Products
CHILTERN HERBS COUNTRY STUFFING	126	5.2	2	23.6	2.3	1.2	0.3	1.0	87.5	Chiltern Herbs
JUST BOUILLON CHICKEN STOCK	9	0.2	0	0.8	0.2	0.5	0.2	1.0	87.5	Kallo Foods
JUST BOUILLON RED MEAT GRAVY	43	2.6	0.8	7.6	0.4	0.2	0.1	1.5	87.5	Kallo Foods
JUST BOUILLON CONCENTRATED STOCK VEGETABLE	35	0.7	0	6	2.4	0.9	0.1	1.5	87.5	Kallo Foods
MARIGOLD SWISS VEGETABLE BOUILLON	243	10.5	0.7	29.4	8.4	8.1	4.0	44.0	37.5	Marigold Health Foods
MERCHANT GOURMET OVEN ROAST TOMATO & POLENTA STUFFING WITH HERBS	175	3	2.8	28	2.1	5.7	3.7	1.1	62.5	Merchant Gourmet
SCHWARTZ RICH ONION GRAVY	24	0.4	0.5	4.3	2.0	0.6	0.5	1.0	87.5	Schwartz
SHROPSHIRE SPICE CO. SAGE & ONION STUFFING MIX	155	6.5	5.6	29.1	2.1	1.4	0.2	0.9	87.5	Shropshire Spice
SIERRA RICA ORGANIC TRADITIONAL CHESTNUT STUFFING	242	6	5.3	49.1	12.4	2.6	0.4	0.5	75.0	Sierra Rica
KNORR CHICKEN STOCK GRANULES	232	13.1	0.4	36.5	31.8	3.7	1.2	44.4	37.5	Unilever
KNORR SIMPLY STOCK CHICKEN	6	1.6	0.1	0.1	0.1	0.0	0.0	0.9	87.5	Unilever
KNORR THE FISH CUBE	7	0.4	0	0.2	0.1	0.5	0.3	0.9	87.5	Unilever

Key

TYPICAL SERVING SIZE: 10G (one stock cube)

All figures are grammes per 100 grammes (expect Energy reading which = Kcal per100 grammes)

Source: The Ethical Company Organisation / The Good Nutrition Guide 2006 - 2008

For explantion of Good Nutrition Guide Score see the "Using the Research Tables" section

THE GOOD NUTRITION GUIDE
WORST CHOICE:

Bisto Favourite Gravy Granules

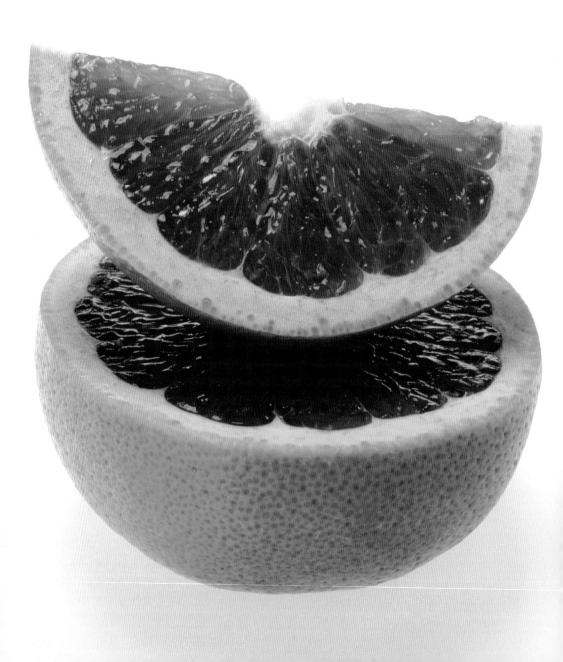

Ice Creams

While the manufacturers are keen to remind us that their products are full of calcium and vitamins A and D, a nutritional defence of ice cream is otherwise pretty difficult to muster. Needless to say, this high fat high sugar dessert is best eaten in moderation: if you're looking to cut down on additives an occasional full-fat indulgence may be better than frequent forays into the reduced fat aisle. For lower calorie, lower sugar alternatives, try fruit sorbets or frozen yoghurts.

ICE CREAM

Ice cream consumption in Britain is the third highest in Europe (behind Denmark and Sweden), at 8 litres per person per year. This may sound like a lot, but it is nothing compared to the Americans, who each manage a hefty 21 litres per year. The proliferation of home freezers has meant that ice cream is no longer an occasional seaside treat but an everyday dessert.

The simplest type of ice cream is made from cream, eggs (or egg yolks) and flavouring such as vanilla essence, fruit or chocolate. The ingredients are whisked together, sieved to make a smooth paste and then frozen until set, with the mixture being stirred regularly to prevent crystals from forming while it freezes. As raw eggs can be a salmonella risk, especially for pregnant women and young children, most commercial ice creams leave them out.

Sorbets are even less complicated than ice cream, and require only fruit puree and ice as their main ingredients. Some may also contain alcohol for flavour, and many are based on sugar syrup, into which fruit and fruit juices are combined. Even so, as sorbets do not contain any milk they are much less fatty than ice creams. The most basic versions, which use fruit sugar for sweetness rather than added sugars, are a particularly good option.

FAT CONTENT

To be labelled as an ice cream a product must contain over 5 per cent fat and over

2.5 per cent milk protein. In "dairy ice creams" this fat must all come from milk, while standard "ice creams" may include fat from sources such as vegetable fat. Many products contain cream as well as milk, which produces a richer texture but increases the saturated fat content. Low fat desserts often use skimmed milk or milk powders in place of cream.

Dairy ice creams may also state that they contain clotted cream, which is over 55 per cent milk fat and the highest in fat of all types of cream. Those that contain extra ingredients such as fudge or brownie pieces are likely to have a particularly high sugar content, and adding wafers and sauces to ice cream will also up the calorie count. While products that describe themselves as "luxury" items are more likely to be high in fat and sugar, this doesn't necessarily mean that non-luxury products are better for you.

ICE CREAM ALTERNATIVES

Frozen yoghurt can be a nutritious alternative to ice cream – it contains the same amount of fat as regular yoghurt and is generally much lower in saturates than other iced desserts. Although it is less readily available than ice cream, most major supermarkets now stock it.

The same is true of soya ice cream, a non-dairy option that is suitable for vegans. This is made with blended soya, and flavoured in the same way as regular ice cream. Soya is lower in fat than cream, although the products may still be high in sugar or sweeteners. If you want to avoid the additives associated with processed foods altogether it is even possible to make your own non-dairy ice cream with soya milk.

Some ice creams are available in individual tubs as well as large containers, which can act as a useful portion guide – or limitation device. If you choose these don't forget to recycle the extra packaging.

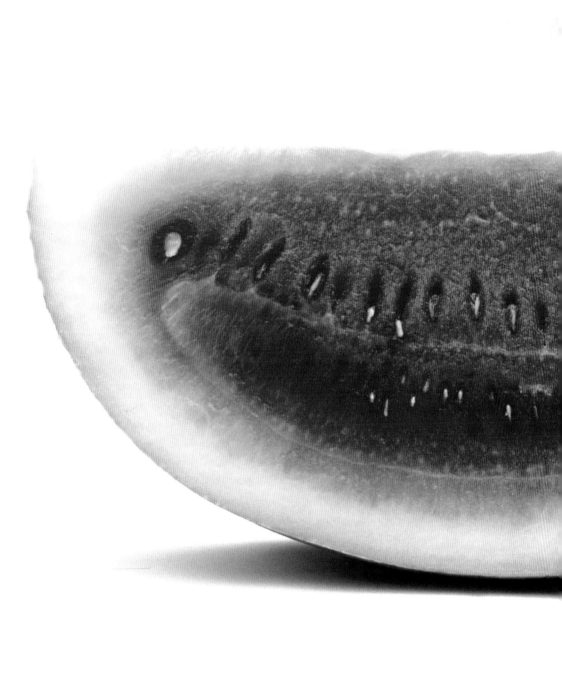

OUR RESEARCH RESULTS

It's clear from the colour scheme in this table that ice creams are all much of a muchness: they are high in sugar, medium in fat, high in saturates and low in salt. While the salt figures are all very similar – either 0.2g or 0.3g per 100g – there is much more variation in the other nutrient categories. Ice creams with cones are inevitably higher in carbohydrates, with the Cornetto Classico and Cornetto Strawberry topping the list at over 30g per 100g. All of the products contain some complex carbohydrates, with the exception of Haagen Dazs Vanilla – in its case the 17.6g of carbohydrates is just sugar.

Nevertheless, Haagen Dazs is not the highest in calories; with 330kcal per 100g, that accolade goes to the Cornetto Classico. The Classico contains more fat (20g per 100g) than any other product surveyed. Lowest in fat are the items in the Dairyland range, each with 8.4g per 100g. They are also lower in saturates, with half the saturated fat of the highest in the survey, Vienetta Mint and Vienetta Vanilla – both of which have 15g. However, at 7.4g out of 8.4g, the level of saturates is proportionally higher in the Dairyland products.

Of the other nutrients, the Cornetto Classico is highest in protein, at 4g per 100g. At 2.6g another Cornetto, Strawberry, is lowest. Both of these – again due to the cone – contain more fibre than the other ice creams in the table. It seems that even within the boundaries of the FSA's categories, there are notable differences between these products – not least a 12g difference between the most and least fatty ice cream surveyed.

THE GOOD NUTRITION GUIDE RECOMMENDS

LOWEST IN SUGARS:
Haagen Dazs Vanilla

LOWEST IN SATURATED FATS:
Dairyland (all products)

LOWEST IN SALT:
Haagen Dazs Vanilla; Mars Ice Cream; Cornetto Strawberry

THE GOOD NUTRITION GUIDE BEST CHOICE:
All products received 37.5 points

BRAND NAME	ENERGY	PROTEIN	FIBRE	CARBOHYDRATES	SUGARS	FAT	SATURATED FAT	SALT	GOOD NUTRITION GUIDE SCORE	Company group
DAIRYLAND RASPBERRY PAVLOVA	187	3.46	0	27.4	19.7	8.4	7.4	0.3	37.5	Dairyland
DAIRYLAND MAPLE & WALNUT	165	2.76	0	20.1	19.7	8.4	7.4	0.3	37.5	Dairyland
DAIRYLAND MINT CHOC CHIP	175	3.12	0	21.2	19.7	8.4	7.4	0.3	37.5	Dairyland
DAIRYLAND RUM & RAISIN	175	3.12	0	21.2	19.7	8.4	7.4	0.3	37.5	Dairyland
DAIRYLAND TOFFEE CRUNCH	187	3.46	0	22.4	19.7	8.4	7.4	0.3	37.5	Dairyland
HAAGEN DAZS VANILLA	223	3.9	0	17.6	17.6	15.2	9.1	0.2	37.5	General Mills
MARS ICE CREAM	281	3.6	0.2	30.1	23.6	16.2	10.6	0.2	37.5	Masterfoods
CORNETTO CLASSICO	330	4.0	1.2	33	24.0	20.0	13.0	0.3	37.5	Unilever
CORNETTO STRAWBERRY	265.0	2.6	0.9	37.0	30.0	12.0	9.3	0.2	37.5	Unilever
VIENETTA MINT	255.0	3.3	0.3	22.0	21.0	17.0	15.0	0.3	37.5	Unilever
VIENETTA VANILLA	252.0	3.3	0.3	22.0	20.0	17.0	15.0	0.3	37.5	Unilever

Key

TYPICAL SERVING SIZE: 100G (two scoops)

All figures are grammes per 100 grammes (expect Energy reading which = Kcal per100 grammes)

Source: The Ethical Company Organisation / The Good Nutrition Guide 2006 - 2008

For explantion of Good Nutrition Guide Score see the "Using the Research Tables" section

THE GOOD NUTRITION GUIDE
WORST CHOICE:

All products received 37.5 points

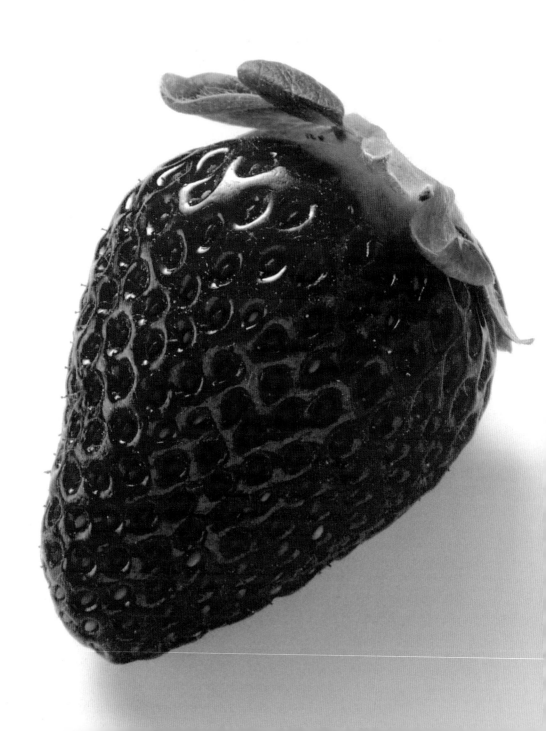

Jams and Spreads

A smear of jam on a slice of toast might not sound like much to worry about, but getting better nutritional (and monetary) value from your spreads could be as simple as switching brands – particularly given that some marmalades are only 20 per cent fruit, while jams and jellies may be bulked up with water. Check the ingredients list to be sure, and try "extra" jams and conserves with a higher fruit content. Or, for a savoury alternative, choose peanut butters made with nuts and nothing else.

JAMS, JELLIES AND MARMALADES

There are strict regulations surrounding the amount of fruit manufacturers have to put in their jams and preserves, but you may be surprised at how little is required. Even in high fruit jams, the sugar content is huge – over 50 per cent – so there's no denying that these popular breakfast items are not the most nutritious thing to spread on your morning toast. Nevertheless, there are substantial differences in fruit and sugar content according to the type of jam you choose, so it's worth knowing which is which.

To be labelled as a "jam", a product must contain at least 35g of fruit pulp or puree per 100g. "Extra jam" must be made up of over 45g of fruit per 100g. These figures are often lower for jams from redcurrants, rosehips, ginger and other more unusual fruits. A "jelly" will be made from fruit juice rather than fruit puree – "extra jelly" will contain more juice or extract than regular jelly. Marmalades can contain a combination of fruit juice, pulp and peel, provided that the overall fruit content is over 20g per 100g.

In nutritional terms, the higher the fruit level the better. Some products will clearly state the amount on the label, but often the information will be hidden in the ingredients list. Jams that get their fruit from pulp or puree are likely to contain more of the nutrients from the fruit, although in all cases the fruit will have been boiled during the production process, which will destroy many of the vital vitamins.

When choosing a reduced sugar jam, be sure that the reduction in sugar has been accompanied by an increase in fruit content, rather than the addition of water. Most low sugar products also require extra gelling agents and preservatives to compensate for the reduction, and may use sweeteners for flavour. Some jams also contain ingredients derived from animals, so may not be suitable for vegetarians.

CHOCOLATE SPREADS

You may think there is nothing nutritionally redeemable about a tub of chocolate spread, but this doesn't stop the manufacturers from suggesting otherwise. A number of companies have been criticised for advertising the vitamin and mineral content of their products while conveniently ignoring the high levels of sugar and fat.

Health claims are not regulated, which means there are no guarantees that a "high calcium" product is otherwise healthy – with chocolate spreads, this is unlikely to be the case. Legislation on this issue is due to be implemented in the next 12 months, but until then consumers need to check

the label to be sure they are not being misled.

PEANUT BUTTER

Some high fat spreads use the fact that they contain less fat than peanut butter as a positive health claim. This may be true in terms of overall fat content, but the real issue is not how much fat is in the product, but what kind of fat appears. Chocolate spreads and similar products are high in unhealthy saturates, but low in monounsaturates and polyunsaturates. The nuts in peanut butter are a rich source of monounsaturated fat, which is one of the "good fats" that many of us need more of in our diets.

While all of these fats – even the healthy ones – should be consumed in moderation, peanut butter is a good alternative to sugary jams and spreads. Many "pure" and organic products are made without any added oils or salt, which makes them a particularly nutritious option. For more variety, try cashew and almond butters or tahini, which is made from sesame seeds.

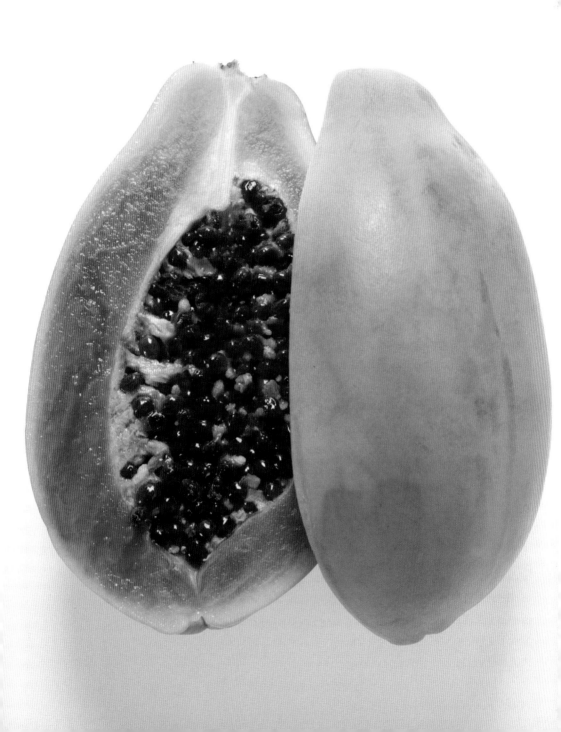

OUR RESEARCH RESULTS

Many of the most popular jams and spreads do not display all eight nutrition figures, which makes it difficult to work out how much sugar, saturated fat and salt they contain. Nevertheless, the small sample collected gives some useful examples of the nutritional value offered by both sweet and savoury spreads. Starting with the savoury options, the two yeast products in the table – Vegemite and Marmite – have similar figures for carbohydrates but differ in nearly every other category. While both products receive green lights for sugars, fats and saturates, Vegemite is slightly lower in sugars and Marmite is lower in fat. Marmite contains more protein and fibre, and also boasts more salt – indeed, with 10.8g per 100g for Marmite and 8.5g for Vegemite, both products are indisputably salty.

Much less salty – although still receiving a red light – is Heinz Sandwich Spread. The Sandwich Spread also gets a red rating for sugars, with a surprisingly high 21.3g. Although low in saturates, it contains a moderate amount of fat overall, at 13.1g per 100g. This is still much lower than Meridian Foods' Crunchy Wholenut Peanut Butter, which has a considerable

48.2g per 100g. While 8.6g of this fat is saturates, the fact that this is a nut-based product means that the remainder will include plenty of beneficial mono- and polyunsaturates.

For the sweet spreads, the main nutrient of interest is sugar, and Robertson's Golden Shred marmalade has plenty – 52.6g per 100g. This is over five times as much as Robertson's Raspberry Jam, which contains just 9.7g of sugar out of a similar number of carbohydrates.

THE GOOD NUTRITION GUIDE RECOMMENDS

LOWEST IN SUGARS:
Marmite

LOWEST IN SATURATED FATS:
Robertson's Golden Shred; Marmite

LOWEST IN SALT:
Robertson's Golden Shred

THE GOOD NUTRITION GUIDE BEST CHOICE:
Robertson's Raspberry Jam

BRAND NAME	ENERGY	PROTEIN	FIBRE	CARBOHYDRATES	SUGARS	FAT	SATURATED FAT	SALT	GOOD NUTRITION GUIDE SCORE	Company group
HEINZ SANDWICH SPREAD	220	0.9	0.6	23.9	21.3	13.1	1.0	2.1	37.5	Heinz
VEGEMITE	191	25.6	0	19.5	1.7	0.9	0.4	8.5	75.0	Kraft
CRUNCHY WHOLENUT PEANUT BUTTER	606	31	6.5	12.1	6.2	48.2	8.6	1.0	25.0	Meridian Foods
ROBERTSON'S GOLDEN SHRED	254	0.2	0.7	62.5	52.6	0.0	0.0	0.0	75.0	Robertson's
ROBERTSON'S RASPBERRY JAM	243	0.6	1.4	59.9	9.7	0.1	0.1	0.1	87.5	Robertson's
MARMITE	219	38.4	3.1	19.2	0.5	0.1	0.0	10.8	75.0	Unilever

Key

TYPICAL SERVING SIZE: 20G (one heaped teaspoon)

All figures are grammes per 100 grammes (expect Energy reading which = Kcal per100 grammes)

Source: The Ethical Company Organisation / The Good Nutrition Guide 2006 - 2008

For explantion of Good Nutrition Guide Score see the "Using the Research Tables" section

THE GOOD NUTRITION GUIDE
WORST CHOICE:

Crunchy Wholenut Peanut Butter

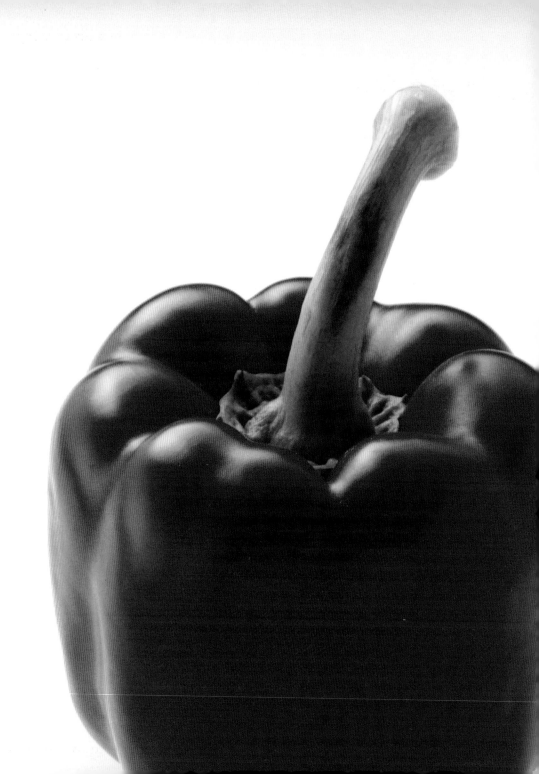

Pasta Sauces

There are few more straightforward meals than pasta and sauce, and with a jar of pasta sauce – or even pasta in sauce – rustling up a plate of hot food becomes even easier. The main concern with supermarket sauces is the level of salt and fat, both of which may be unexpectedly high in some products. The ingredients list will reveal the amount of added vegetables in the sauce (the more the better), and whether it is made with water, concentrate or tomato purée.

SHOP-BOUGHT OR HOME-MADE?

The best way to see how well shop-bought pasta sauce compares with home-made is to look at the ingredients list. In some cases, the key ingredients may be missing in the processed version. Spaghetti carbonara, for example, is usually made with eggs and bacon, but pre-prepared sauces will often use diced ham and leave out the eggs altogether. Eggs contain all of the essential amino acids needed in a balanced diet, so the loss of this protein reduces the overall nutritional value of the dish. If the richness of the eggs has been reproduced with cream, the carbonara will also be higher in fat.

Most of the sauces available use tomatoes as the main ingredient. For a higher concentration of nutrients, pick sauces that contain just tomatoes or tomatoes with tomato puree, and which are not diluted with water. Vegetable sauces will usually include extra mushrooms and peppers, but check how much is actually present – in some cases the proportions may be very small. Be aware that over-cooking can reduce the number of vitamins in vegetables; adding your own at home may be a healthier option.

One ingredient that probably won't appear in home-made pasta sauces is modified maize starch. This is a thickener used in many processed products. The term "modified" does not refer to genetic modification – although in future this may be the case – but to chemical or physical processing that allows the starch to survive industrial use.

HIDDEN INGREDIENTS

Processed foods such as pasta sauces are a prominent source of salt in many diets. This so-called "hidden" salt is a problem because most of us aren't even aware that we're eating it – particularly if it's found in a product that we wouldn't automatically associate with high salt levels. Most jars of sauce are already seasoned, so don't be tempted to add more at home.

Carbonaras and "creamy" sauces may be high in fat if they are made with fresh cream or butter. Some also include hydrogenated oil, which is a source of trans fats. If you regularly use pasta sauces, pick tomato-based products more often than cream-based ones, as there could be more than 10g of extra fat in the latter. Many sauces also contain added sugar and glucose syrup, so look out for these on the label.

Quick cook products, such as microwaveable pouches, may contain more additives than heat-on-the-hob options. Products containing cream, in particular, often require extra stabilisers and emulsifiers to prevent them from separating during the cooking process.

ALTERNATIVES

Pesto is another alternative to pasta sauce. Made from basil, pine nuts, parmesan and olive oil, it has a strong flavour and is used in much smaller quantities (less than a tablespoon for a one-person dish) than most ready-made sauces. Pesto is very high in fat, but if olive oil has been used a significant amount of this will be the less unhealthy monounsaturated variety. Most supermarket pestos don't include parmesan cheese, which will have an effect on their fat and salt content.

For a less processed choice of pasta sauce try passata, which is made from tomatoes that have been cooked and sieved to remove the pips. Authentic passata (which is available from many organic food shops) contains no added ingredients, and can be used on its own or as a base for meat or vegetables.

OUR RESEARCH RESULTS

In the Pasta Sauces table, Dolmio Light lives up to its name as the product with

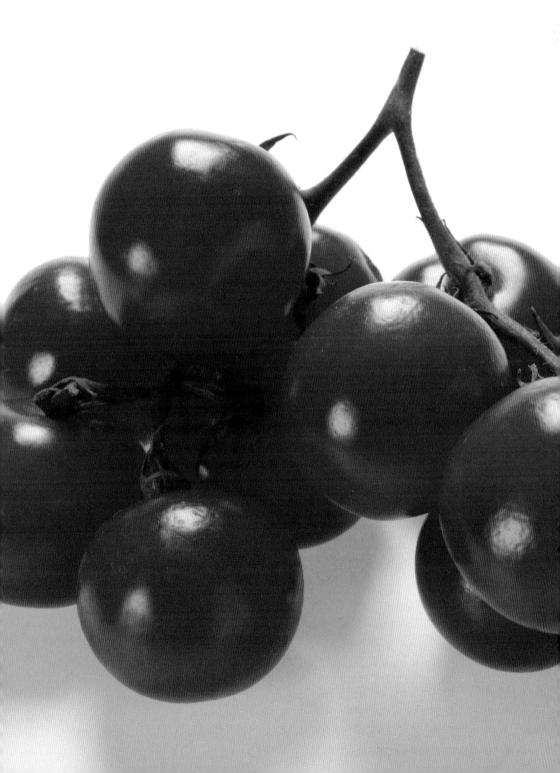

the most green lights under the FSA's system. It contains none of the oil found in many pasta sauces, so scores 0.1 for fat and a resounding 0 for saturates. Dolmio Original and Bertolli Tomato and Basil are not far behind at 0.2g and 0.1g for saturates. The Seeds Of Change option, on the other hand, contains a significantly higher 14g of fat. The survey displays a clear distinction between sauces based upon tomatoes, those based upon cream and those that use pesto-style oils. While Seeds of Change's Sundried Tomato & Basil (containing olive oil) has a particularly high fat content, it has a much lower saturates level than Loyd Grossman's Carbonara and Tomato & Mascarpone sauces, both of which use dairy products amongst their ingredients.

When it comes to salt, only Seeds of Change receives a red light with 1.8g per 100g. The rest contain a moderate amount of salt within a small range of 0.9 to 1.2g. There is a similarly limited range in the carbohydrates figures, which all fall between 6.8 and 9.2g per 100g. Not so for sugars: here, the products show considerable differences, with Loyd Grossman Carbonara on a slight 0.6g per 100g while Dolmio Original and others contain over 6g. What the figures cannot say is how much of this can be attributed to added sugars.

Of the remaining categories, Seeds of Change has the highest figure for fibre, and two Loyd Grossman sauces, Carbonara and Tomato & Mascarpone, are at the top of the list for protein. The two with the most amber and red ratings, Loyd Grossman Tomato & Mascarpone and Seeds of Change Sundried Tomato & Basil are also the highest in calories. The product with the highest score overall – and the lowest total number of calories – is Dolmio Original Light.

THE GOOD NUTRITION GUIDE RECOMMENDS

LOWEST IN SUGARS:
Loyd Grossman Carbonara

LOWEST IN SATURATED FATS:
Dolmio Original Light

LOWEST IN SALT:
Loyd Grossman Puttanesca; Loyd Grossman Carbonara; Loyd Grossman Tomato & Mascarpone; Bertolli Tomato & Basil

BRAND NAME	ENERGY	PROTEIN	FIBRE	CARBOHYDRATES	SUGARS	FAT	SATURATED FAT	SALT	GOOD NUTRITION GUIDE SCORE	Company group
LOYD GROSSMAN PUTTANESCA	90	1.7	0.9	6.8	6.2	6.2	0.8	0.9	62.5	Chivers Hartley
LOYD GROSSMAN CARBONARA	123	2.8	0.1	7.5	0.6	9.1	5.6	0.9	50.0	Chivers Hartley
LOYD GROSSMAN TOMATO & MASCARPONE	138	2.3	1.1	9	5.5	7.4	6.1	0.9	37.5	Chivers Hartley
DOLMIO ORIGINAL	53	1.3	0.8	9.2	6.1	1.2	0.2	1.1	75.0	Masterfoods
DOLMIO ORIGINAL LIGHT	37	1.2	0.7	7.8	4.7	0.1	0.0	1.2	87.5	Masterfoods
SEEDS OF CHANGE SUNDRIED TOMATO & BASIL	168	1.6	1.2	9	6.7	14.0	2.0	1.8	37.5	Seeds Of Change
BERTOLLI TOMATO & BASIL	43	1.2	0.4	7.3	6.2	1.0	0.1	0.9	87.5	Unilever

Key

TYPICAL SERVING SIZE: 150G (1/3 of a jar)

All figures are grammes per 100 grammes (expect Energy reading which = Kcal per100 grammes)

Source: The Ethical Company Organisation / The Good Nutrition Guide 2006 - 2008

For explantion of Good Nutrition Guide Score see the "Using the Research Tables" section

THE GOOD NUTRITION GUIDE
BEST CHOICE:
Dolmio Original Light

THE GOOD NUTRITION GUIDE
WORST CHOICE:
Loyd Grossman Tomato & Mascarpone;
Seeds Of Change Sundried Tomato & Basil

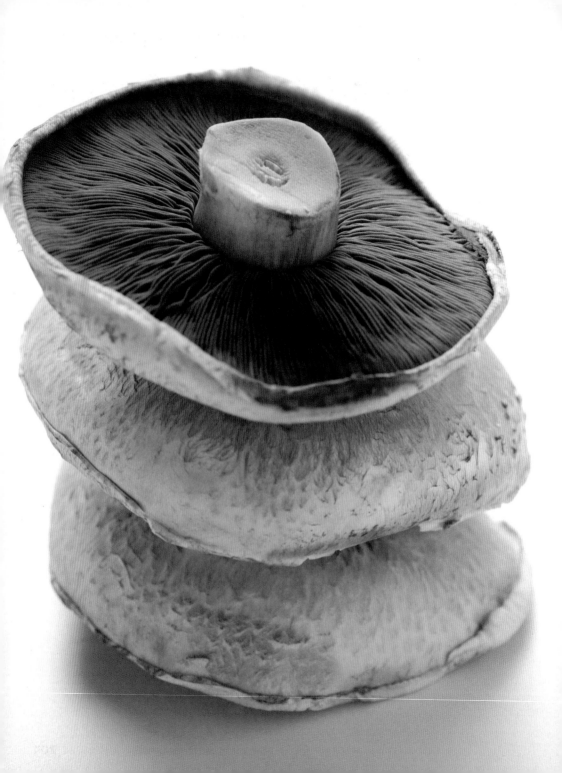

Pasties and Savoury Snacks

Folklore states that a proper Cornish pasty should be tough enough to survive falling down a mine shaft, but it's unlikely many of today's less resilient snacks would pass the test. While a traditional pasty, stuffed with good quality steak and vegetables, is the pinnacle of nutritious fast food, some of the mass-produced imitations contain much cheaper meat and thin, fatty pastry. Even more worryingly, some of them may contain as much salt as five bags of Walkers Ready Salted crisps.

CORNISH PASTIES

Pasties originated in the tin mines of Cornwall, where workers needed a healthy and filling meal to take with them underground. With meat and vegetables at one end, fruit at the other, and a thick pastry rind for holding onto with dirty hands, the pasty was an ideal practical and nutritional solution. The idea caught on, and pasties still appear in the savoury snacks section of most supermarkets – but are their nutritional credentials as good as they were 100 years ago?

Mass-produced pasties generally use puff pastry. This is lighter than short crust pastry, but as some recipes call for equal amounts of butter and flour, it can be very high in fat. Short crust pastry is usually baked with half butter to flour, making it potentially a healthier option. Pasties made with a thicker layer of short crust pastry will be higher in carbohydrates, and are usually much more filling.

Cornish pasties are made with beef, potatoes, onions and occasionally swede. Supermarket versions will nearly always cut down on the more expensive beef in favour of extra vegetables such as potatoes and carrots. Indeed, potato is frequently listed as the main ingredient by weight. Better quality pasties will use diced steak rather than mince, and contain a higher proportion of meat as a whole. Most vegetarian products are also based on potato, usually with added cheese and onion.

High in Fat and Salt

Both the meat and vegetable-based products are usually high in saturated fats, with most having much more than the Food Standards Agency's "high" rating of 5g saturates per 100g. Like many processed products, pasties can also be exceptionally high in salt, with some providing almost half of the government's guideline daily allowance of 6g in one serving. At the moment, none of the mainstream companies offer reduced fat or salt alternatives for their most popular products.

A major difference between traditional pasties and the ones sold by the supermarkets is that the latter are often sold as snacks – to be eaten between meals – rather than as a main meal in themselves. When the products in question contain over half the recommended daily intake of salt and fat, this is of particular concern.

Pork Pies and Other Snacks

Alongside the pasties are numerous other savoury snacks such as pork pies and Scotch eggs. While both are inherently fatty foods – due in part to the layer of pork jelly in the former and fried breadcrumbs in the latter, as well as the meat content – their nutritional value varies greatly according to the quality of the ingredients. Scotch eggs in particular have gained a reputation for using cheap sausage meat, which is usually revealed in the low percentage of meat given on the label.

In pork pies the main difference is between the cured meats used by mass-produced pies and the uncured pork favoured by smaller butchers. If the curing process involves the addition of salt, this will be reflected in the sodium content of the pie. The pastry for pork pies is typically made with lard from animal fat, which has become less popular in home cooking since healthier vegetable fats have been made available. Although lard does not contain trans fats, it is full of cholesterol-raising saturates.

Our Research Results

It's worth remembering with most of the pasties in the table that a serving is likely to be much more than 100g – double or more in the case of the Ginsters products. This means that even though the pasty

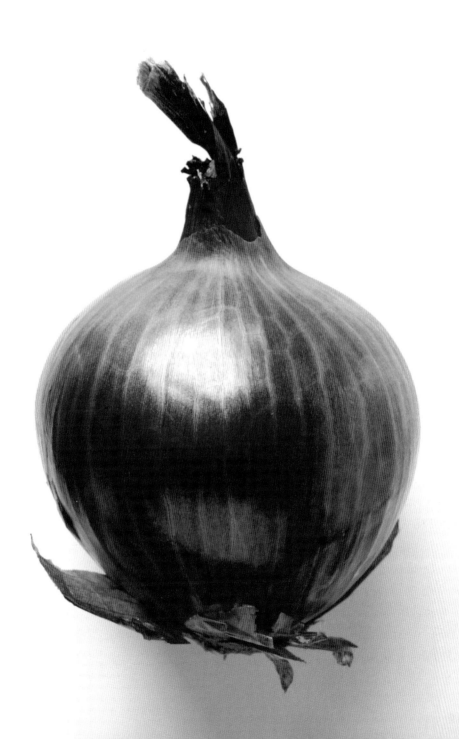

may receive an amber or green rating for a certain nutrient, the amount consumed per serving will actually be much higher. So a pasty that contains 1.5g of salt per 100g (such as the Quorn Mince & Onion Slice) may have up to, or even more than, 3g of salt per serving – that's half the recommended daily intake. The least salty product in the table, Ginsters' Peppered Steak Slice, contains 0.7g salt per 100g, which is equivalent to 1.3g per slice.

Equally concerning are the figures for fats. None of the products surveyed have a green rating for this nutrient. The Quorn Mince & Onion Slice has the lowest fat content with 11.7g per 100g. Ginsters Peppered Steak Slice and Ready To Eat Five Cornish Rolls both have a red rating, containing 20.3 and 20.9g per 100g respectively. The saturates figures are even higher: five products have a red rating, three of which contain 9g or more per 100g. Assuming a typical serving of 200g, the Ginsters Chicken & Mushroom Slice, Ginsters Peppered Steak Slice and Ready To Eat Five Cornish Rolls contain the equivalent of just under an entire day's recommended intake of saturates.

Overall, sugars are a less prominent nutrient in these products – with one exception. Apart from Maggi Hot Pockets, all of the pasties contain 2.3g or less of sugars per 100g, which earns them a green rating from the FSA. The Maggi snack has a much higher figure – 11.4g per 100g, a whole 9g above the next highest, Quorn Mince & Onion Slice. Notably, amongst the four other nutrients, the meat-free Quorn slice is lowest in protein, while Ginsters Peppered Steak Slice is highest.

THE GOOD NUTRITION GUIDE RECOMMENDS

LOWEST IN SUGARS:
Ginsters Peppered Steak Slice

LOWEST IN SATURATED FATS:
Quorn Mince & Onion Slice

LOWEST IN SALT:
Ginsters Peppered Steak Slice

THE GOOD NUTRITION GUIDE BEST CHOICE:
Quorn Mince & Onion Slice

BRAND NAME	ENERGY	PROTEIN	FIBRE	CARBOHYDRATES	SUGARS	FAT	SATURATED FAT	SALT	GOOD NUTRITION GUIDE SCORE	Company group
GINSTERS CHICKEN & MUSHROOM SLICE	259.0	7.5	1.7	18.2	1.4	17.3	9.5	0.9	50.0	Ginsters
GINSTERS ORIGINAL CORNISH PASTY	255.0	6.2	1.9	21.6	1.3	15.5	7.5	1.3	50.0	Ginsters
GINSTERS PEPPER SLICE	285.0	9.5	3.2	16.1	1.2	20.3	9.9	0.7	37.5	Ginsters
MAGGI HOT POCKETS TWO CRISPY PASTY, CHEESE & TOMATO	282.0	8.0	2.0	26.9	11.4	15.8	5.5	0.7	37.5	Maggi
QUORN MINCE & ONION SLICE	226.0	5.6	4.5	24.5	2.3	11.7	5.0	1.5	62.5	Marlow Foods
READY TO EAT FIVE CORNISH ROLLS	301.0	7.0	4.6	21.2	1.5	20.9	9.0	1.3	37.5	Pork Farms

Key

TYPICAL SERVING SIZE: 200G (one pasty)

All figures are grammes per 100 grammes (expect Energy reading which = Kcal per 100 grammes)

Source: The Ethical Company Organisation / The Good Nutrition Guide 2006 - 2008

For explanation of Good Nutrition Guide Score see the "Using the Research Tables" section

THE GOOD NUTRITION GUIDE
WORST CHOICE:

Ginsters Peppered Steak Slice; Maggi Hot
Pockets Cheese & Tomato; Ready To Eat
Five Cornish Rolls

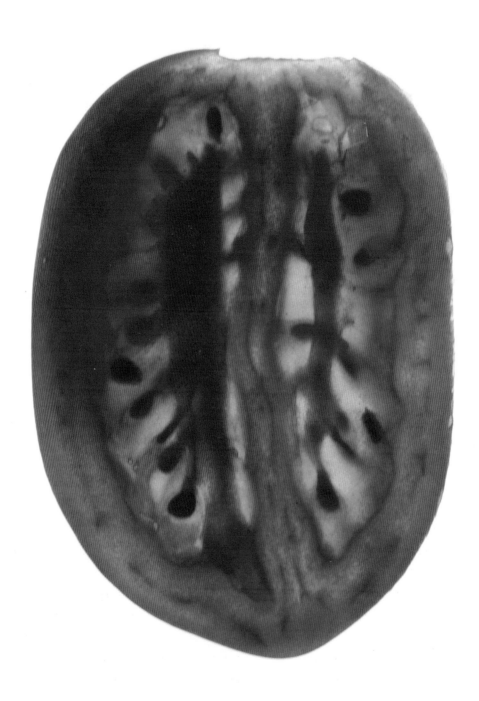

Pizza

There are few food categories in which there is more choice than pizza: chilled or frozen, thin or thick crust, veggie or meat – that's not to mention calzones, pizza baguettes, microwave slices and make-it-yourself kits. Any pizza that contains a thick bread base, thin layer of cheese, plenty of vegetable topping and a small quantity of meat or fish will provide a good variety of nutrients – but be sure to find out whether these include large quantities of fat, sugar and salt.

BALANCE OF GOOD HEALTH

The Food Standards Agency uses a pizza to illustrate the principle behind its Balance of Good Health guide. This shows how the proportions of carbohydrate, fat, protein and other nutrients can be balanced as part of a good diet. Using ready-made pizza as an example, it shows how a pizza is mostly bread and cereals (the base), with milk and dairy (cheese), vegetables (tomato paste) and meat, fish or alternatives (the topping). Picking a pizza that combines all of these elements will help to ensure that it is providing a full range of ingredients from all the food groups.

There should be little nutritional difference between chilled and frozen pizzas although, like chilled ready meals, the refrigerated varieties might contain extra additives and preservatives. The biggest distinction between brands will be the extra ingredients, and whether the pizza topping is thin or deep fill. If a company produces both chilled and frozen varieties it may be helpful to compare the two.

PIZZA BASES

The Balance of Good Health recommends choosing thick crust pizzas over thin crust, because these will provide more of their energy from the carbohydrates contained in the bread base. Thin crust pizzas could be eaten with extra bread to increase their carbohydrate content, but opt for a crusty roll rather than buttery garlic bread, which would increase the amount of fat in the meal.

If possible pick pizza bases made with wholemeal flour. Unlike white flour, wholemeal contains the outer parts of the grain, making it much higher in fibre – an essential nutrient for a healthy digestive system. Wholemeal bases are often sold separately, allowing you to add your own cheese and topping at home. This may be a good idea if you are looking for a quick-cook alternative to supermarket oven pizza.

Stuffed crust pizzas are mostly available at pizza restaurants. These contain an extra layer of cheese in the base or sides of the pizza, and as a result will be much higher in fat than a standard thick-crust option. The fat content may also vary according to the amount of water in the mozzarella or the alternative type of cheese used – many will also contain cheaper cheddars. Vegetarians will need to check whether the cheese has been made with animal rennet.

TOPPINGS

Some of the most famous pizza toppings – olives, pepperoni and anchovies – are high salt foods, indicating that they contain a lot of sodium. While this doesn't mean they should always be avoided, it may be worth trying different toppings if you are concerned about your salt intake. "Meat feast" toppings, containing sausage, mince and pepperoni, are likely to be high in saturated fat.

Added toppings such as these are subject to specific labelling regulations, which means that the company may not have to tell you what's in them. If an ingredient makes up less than 25 per cent of the overall product, its own ingredients don't have to be revealed on the label – so it may not be possible to find out how many additives have gone into the pepperoni on your pizza.

Pizza-makers Goodfellas note on their website that their pizzas "do not, as yet, supply one portion of fruit and vegetables" according to the government's five-a-day guidelines – even including the tomato topping. This is likely to be the case for most manufacturers, but even a few sliced peppers or onion pieces makes a difference to the nutritional content. Adding extra fruit and vegetables (such as courgette, sweetcorn or pineapple) at home will

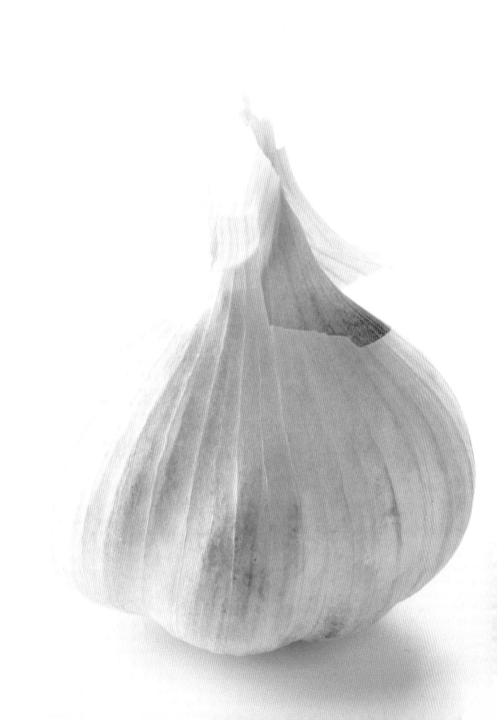

improve the balance. Another way to get more vegetables into the meal is to serve the pizza with a side salad of mixed leaves and tomatoes.

OUR RESEARCH RESULTS

There is a lot of orange in the Pizzas table, with the majority of the products receiving moderate ratings for fat, saturates and salt. It appears that there is very little difference between the frozen and chilled products surveyed; both have similar ratings for all of the major nutrients, and there are no obvious trends in the individual figures that would allow for any general statements about the two groups. It is, however, possible to observe that there are more red lights for saturates in the frozen pizzas section of the table, and that the higher fat products (Chicago Town Deep Dish Pepperoni Pizza, 14.8g; Goodfella's Chicken & Pesto, 11.8g and Goodfella's Loaded Cheese, 11.5g) are also all frozen.

For all of the products, chilled and frozen, the salt content falls between 1 and 1.5g per 100g, which could work out at as much as 6g per whole pizza. While there is only a small amount of variation in carbohydrates levels across the table, the figures for sugar are more diverse. Against an average figure of 3.7g per 100g, Goodfella's Chicken & Pesto and Trancio Margherita Deep & Crispy stand out with 5.2 and 6.0g of sugar – both enough to get them a moderate rating for this nutrient. There is also a wide range for calories, from the Pizza Express Sloppy Giusseppe at 191kcal per 100g to the Chicago Town Deep Dish Pepperoni Pizza at 302kcal.

THE GOOD NUTRITION GUIDE RECOMMENDS

LOWEST IN SUGARS:
Goodfella's Loaded Cheese (Frozen)

LOWEST IN SATURATED FATS:
Pizza Express La Reine

LOWEST IN SALT:
Goodfella's Loaded Cheese (Frozen); Grande Cucina Pepperoni Pizzas (Frozen); The Pizza Company Thin & Crispy Cheese & Tomato Pizza

Brand Name	Energy	Protein	Fibre	Carbohydrates	Sugars	Fat	Saturated Fat	Salt	Good Nutrition Guide Score	Company group
Chicago Town Deep Dish Pepperoni Pizza (Frozen)	302.0	12.1	1.9	30.1	2.5	14.8	7.0	1.3	50.0	Chicago Town
Five Cheese Pan Pizza To Go (Frozen)	292.0	11.8	1.8	39.4	2.8	9.7	5.9	1.5	50.0	Chicago Town
Goodfella's Chicken & Pesto (Frozen)	257.0	10.8	2.4	26.9	5.2	11.8	2.7	1.3	50.0	Green Isle Foods
Goodfella's Loaded Cheese (Frozen)	261.0	12.5	2.1	26.8	2.1	11.5	6.0	1.0	50.0	Green Isle Foods
Grande Cucina Pepperoni Pizzas (Frozen)	220.0	10.8	5.5	25.2	4.7	8.4	4.5	1.0	62.5	Little Big Food Company
Trancio Margherita Deep & Crispy (Frozen)	228.0	8.3	2.5	29.4	6.0	8.6	4.3	1.3	50.0	Little Big Food Company
Pizza Express American	233.0	11.5	2.4	27.7	3.3	8.5	3.6	1.3	62.5	Pizza Express
Pizza Express American Hot	221.0	11.0	3.5	27.3	3.8	7.6	3.3	1.3	62.5	Pizza Express
Pizza Express La Reine	193.0	10.2	2.7	25.0	3.4	5.8	2.2	1.3	62.5	Pizza Express
Pizza Express Margherita	208.0	10.1	2.4	28.5	3.7	6.0	3.1	1.3	62.5	Pizza Express
Pizza Express Quattro Formaggi	243.0	12.1	2.3	26.5	3.6	9.8	5.3	1.5	50.0	Pizza Express
Pizza Express Sloppy Giusseppe	191.0	9.4	2.5	24.1	3.9	6.3	2.7	1.3	62.5	Pizza Express
The Pizza Company Thin & Crispy Cheese & Tomato Pizza	260.0	11.4	2.2	33.3	3.6	9.0	5.3	1.0	50.0	The Pizza Company

Key

TYPICAL SERVING SIZE: 200G (half a pizza)

All figures are grammes per 100 grammes (expect Energy reading which = Kcal per100 grammes)

Source: The Ethical Company Organisation / The Good Nutrition Guide 2006 - 2008

For explantion of Good Nutrition Guide Score see the "Using the Research Tables" section

THE GOOD NUTRITION GUIDE
BEST CHOICE:

Grande Cucina Pepperoni Pizzas (Frozen);
Pizza Express American; Pizza Express
American Hot; Pizza Express La Reine;
Pizza Express Margherita; Pizza Express
Sloppy Giusseppe

THE GOOD NUTRITION GUIDE
WORST CHOICE:

All remaining products receive 50 points

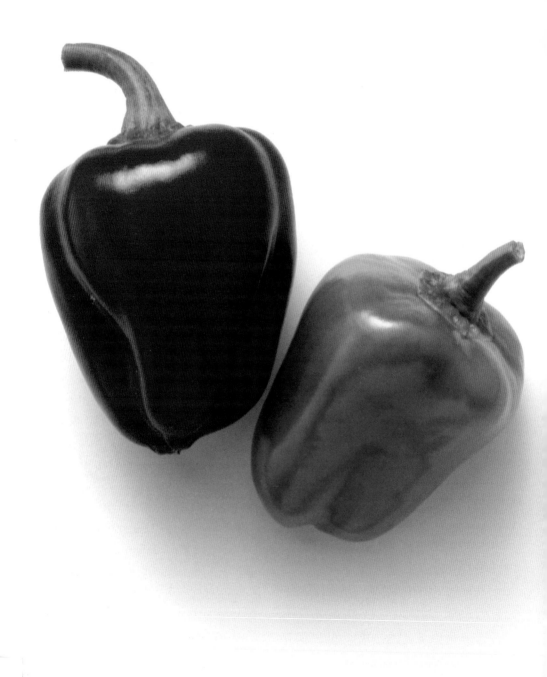

Quiche

Whether it's for a main meal or a lunchtime snack, quiches are a great alternative to fast food. But with their crumbly pastry and creamy egg and cheese centre, they are always going to be high in fat. Still, there is plenty of scope for finding the best nutritional options: for a lower-fat version, choose products that contain less cheese and no added cream, and stick to a small slice of a bigger flan (complete with a side order of vegetables) rather than a whole individual quiche.

OWN BRANDS

Most supermarket quiches are own brands, meaning that your choice of product is restricted to wherever you do your shopping. With no competition from external brands, supermarkets are in close contest with one another for the best prices, which some have claimed can lead to reduced quality foods. Joanna Blythman reports in her book Shopped that suppliers for the major chains have complained of being forced to lower the quality of their raw materials in order to keep up with ever-decreasing prices in-store.

There is often a significant difference in fat, sugar and salt content between the luxury, mid-range and budget options, so how much you choose to spend could have an impact on the nutritional value of the product. Nevertheless, it is very difficult to tell from the packaging whether the standard of ingredients is significantly better in "best" range products. Terms such as "vintage" or "traditional" mean little in terms of nutrition, so the most useful indicator of quality may be the ingredients list, which will show ingredient percentages and the number of additives present.

Crucially, it is not always the case that the more expensive option is healthier; sometimes the number of additives is just as high in the more complicated, upmarket products as in the simple budget varieties. There is also a fine line between "luxury" and "indulgent": most of the extra cost of a pricier quiche may go towards augmenting it with rich cheese and cream, which will vastly increase its fat content. While it would be reasonable to assume that quiches – as a savoury food – are relatively low in sugar, many contain added sugars such as glucose syrup and dextrose.

QUICHE LORRAINE

Probably the most well known type of quiche is the quiche Lorraine, which was originally popularised in the Lorraine region of France. It is traditionally made with a short-crust pastry base, filled with eggs, Swiss cheese and bacon. A good quality supermarket version of the dish should follow this recipe, but many use cheaper substitutes such as cheddar for the Swiss cheese. Check the label to see how much meat is actually contained in the quiche; it may be very little. Current labelling regulations mean that the company will not be obliged to list any added ingredients in the bacon if it makes up less than 25 per cent of the product overall.

Like other quiches, some variations on the quiche Lorraine use cream. The amount of fat contained in the added cream will have an effect on the overall figure for the quiche. While single cream is better for you than double cream, crème fraîche and whipping cream may be just as high in fat. Other fats will be found in the pastry, which could contain trans fats as well as saturates if it has been made with hydrogenated margarine. Although the addition of vegetables may make the vegetarian options appear healthier, the presence of extra cheese means they are frequently higher in fat – this is particularly true of the three cheese and cheese and onion versions.

INDIVIDUAL AND FULL-SIZE QUICHES

While the supermarkets recommend that a serving is quarter of a standard 350g-400g quiche, it is usually tempting to eat half – or more – as a main meal. A good way to increase the nutrient content of this meal may be to have a smaller slice of quiche with a serving of brown bread and side salad, or with boiled new potatoes and vegetables. Choose a quiche that already contains vegetables, as these will contribute towards a serving from this food group.

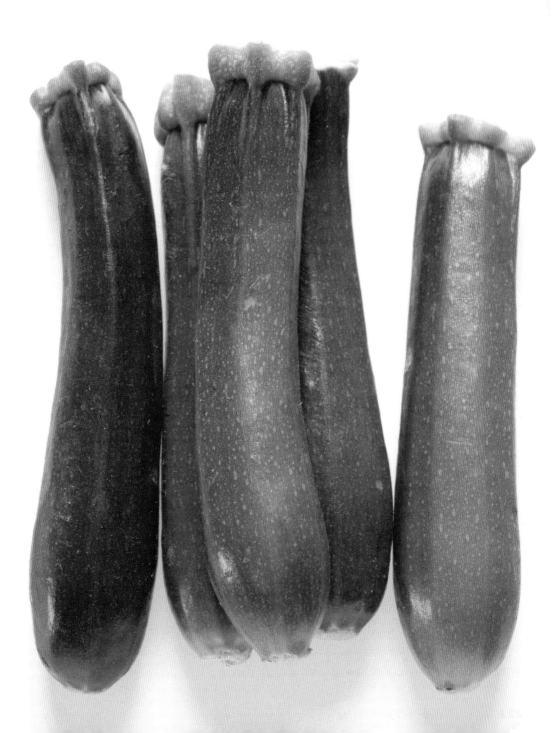

OUR RESEARCH RESULTS

Quiche may be an intrinsically fatty food, but the table suggests that we should perhaps be more concerned about its saturates content than the overall amount of fat. Across all of the supermarket brands, there are many more red ratings for saturates than there are for fat, with only six out of 39 products receiving a moderate rating for saturates. Highest in fat are Morrisons Cheese & Onion quiche at 21.8g per 100g and Asda Extra Special Wensleydale & Tomato at 21.1g. The Asda Extra Special Wensleydale & Tomato is also the highest in saturates, with 13.2g per 100g, followed by Asda Extra Special Quiche Lorraine at 12.2g.

The majority of the quiches surveyed fall into the moderate category for salt content, the highest figure in the table being Sainsbury's Quiche Lorraine with 1.1g per 100g. Others, including Asda's Chicken & Mushroom and Good For You Cheese & Onion have a much lower figure of 0.3g per 100g. Amongst the remaining nutrients, all of the products have a low rating for sugars, with Morrisons' Roasted Root Vegetable quiche displaying the highest figure of just 4.5g per 100g. This quiche is also packed with more fibre than any other in the table – 6.9g per 100g.

THE GOOD NUTRITION GUIDE RECOMMENDS

LOWEST IN SUGARS:
Asda Chicken & Mushroom; Morrisons Smoked Ham, Cheese, Chicken & Leek Flan

LOWEST IN SATURATED FATS:
Morrisons Eat Smart Reduced Fat Quiche Lorraine

LOWEST IN SALT:
Asda Chicken & Mushroom; Asda Good For You Cheese & Onion; Asda Spinach & Ricotta; Morrisons Eat Smart Reduced Fat Cheese & Onion

BEST CHOICE:
Asda Good For You Cheese & Onion; Morrisons Eat Smart Reduced Fat Cheese & Onion

WORST CHOICE:
Asda Extra Special Wensleydale & Tomato; Morrisons Cheese & Onion; Sainsbury's Quiche Lorraine; Tesco Cheese & Bacon

Brand Name	Energy	Protein	Fibre	Carbohydrates	Sugars	Fat	Saturated Fat	Salt	Good Nutrition Guide Score	Company group
Bacon & Leek	245	7.3	1.9	17.4	1.9	16.2	8.0	0.7	50.0	Asda
Cheese & Onion	266	10.5	2.5	16.5	1.7	17.5	8.9	0.6	50.0	Asda
Chicken & Mushroom	247	8.7	2	18.5	1.3	15.4	7.4	0.3	62.5	Asda
Extra Special Davistow Cheddar & Caramelised Onion	287	5.4	2	22.1	2.3	19.7	11.2	0.6	50.0	Asda
Extra Special Quiche Lorraine	266	7.8	2.3	19.1	2.2	17.6	12.2	0.9	50.0	Asda
Extra Special Somerset Brie & Bacon	261	6.6	3	19.5	2.2	17.4	10.3	0.8	50.0	Asda
Extra Special Wensleydale & Tomato	294	6.5	2.1	19.4	2.5	21.1	13.2	0.7	37.5	Asda
Good For You Cheese & Onion	208	10.9	4.2	20	2.1	9.4	4.0	0.3	75.0	Asda
Quiche Lorraine	246	6.6	4.2	18.5	1.9	16.2	7.8	0.7	50.0	Asda
Spinach & Ricotta	247	6.8	1.8	18.7	1.5	16.1	7.9	0.3	62.5	Asda
Tomato, Sausage & Bacon	237	7.9	2.5	18.2	1.9	14.7	6.8	0.8	50.0	Asda
Broccoli	248	8	3.2	17.1	2.8	16.4	8.2	0.7	50.0	Morrisons
Cheese & Onion	300	8.8	1.4	17.2	2.3	21.8	10.4	1.0	37.5	Morrisons
Eat Smart Reduced Fat Cheese & Onion	226	9.5	2.2	23.5	2.7	10.5	4.5	0.3	75.0	Morrisons
Eat Smart Reduced Fat Quiche Lorraine	209	9.4	0.5	17.8	2.3	9.8	3.3	0.7	62.5	Morrisons
Mediterranean Style	241	4.9	1.6	18.2	3.0	16.5	7.1	0.5	50.0	Morrisons
Smoked Ham, Cheese, Chicken & Leek Flan	262	6.9	0.9	20.7	1.3	16.8	3.8	0.7	62.5	Morrisons
Squash & Ricotta	286	6.1	1.8	23.8	2.2	18.5	8.3	0.6	50.0	Morrisons
Tomato, Bacon & Mushroom	251	6.2	1.3	17.9	2.7	17.2	7.5	0.8	50.0	Morrisons
Quiche Lorraine Quiche Lorraine	245	7.4	2	18.4	1.5	15.7	7.0	0.8	50.0	Morrisons
Roasted Root Vegetable	236	6.2	6.9	16	4.5	16.3	7.6	0.8	50.0	Morrisons
The Best Quiche Lorraine	240	9.3	2.1	19.2	3.4	14.0	7.6	0.8	50.0	Morrisons
The Best Vintage Cheddar & Onion	244.0	5.1	1.9	21.0	3.7	15.5	8.3	0.5	50.0	Morrisons
Broccoli, Tomato & Cheese	203.0	5.2	2.3	16.9	2.5	12.9	3.8	0.6	62.5	Sainsbury's
Cheese & Onion	287.0	9.6	3.7	20.5	2.1	18.5	6.5	0.6	50.0	Sainsbury's
Quiche Lorraine	303.0	10.6	4.0	19.5	1.9	20.3	7.6	1.1	37.5	Sainsbury's
Sausage, Tomato & Bacon	247.0	6.6	2.2	17.4	3.0	16.8	5.2	1.0	50.0	Sainsbury's
Spinach & Ricotta	223.0	5.0	1.4	19.4	2.0	13.9	4.1	0.5	62.5	Sainsbury's
Broccoli	250.0	6.0	1.4	17.6	3.5	15.5	7.6	0.5	50.0	Tesco
Cheese & Bacon	295.0	8.0	1.1	17.7	2.6	17.2	9.2	0.5	37.5	Tesco
Cheese & Onion	285.0	7.7	1.3	17.9	3.3	21.2	9.5	0.8	50.0	Tesco
Deep Filled Pepper, Goats' Cheese & Red Pesto	259.0	7.0	1.4	17.0	2.6	19.8	8.7	0.5	50.0	Tesco
Quiche Lorraine	280.0	8.0	1.2	17.5	3.4	18.1	8.4	1.0	50.0	Tesco
Broccoli & Gruyere	244.0	8.2	1.7	15.4	2.1	19.5	7.4	0.5	50.0	Waitrose
Buttered Leek	254.0	6.8	1.4	16.5	2.7	16.6	7.8	0.5	50.0	Waitrose
Farmhouse Cheddar & Onion	257.0	8.1	1.3	15.4	2.6	17.9	8.3	0.6	50.0	Waitrose
Quiche Lorraine	272.0	8.5	1.7	16.0	1.8	18.1	7.8	0.7	50.0	Waitrose
Spinach & Ricotta	239.0	6.7	1.3	16.4	2.3	19.3	6.9	0.5	50.0	Waitrose
Wiltshire Ham, Tomato & Cheddar	229.0	8.1	1.4	14.9	2.5	16.3	6.8	0.5	50.0	Waitrose

Key

Typical serving size: 100g (quarter of a quiche)

All figures are grammes per 100 grammes (expect Energy reading which = Kcal per100 grammes)

Source: The Ethical Company Organisation / The Good Nutrition Guide 2006 - 2008

For explantion of Good Nutrition Guide Score see the "Using the Research Tables" section

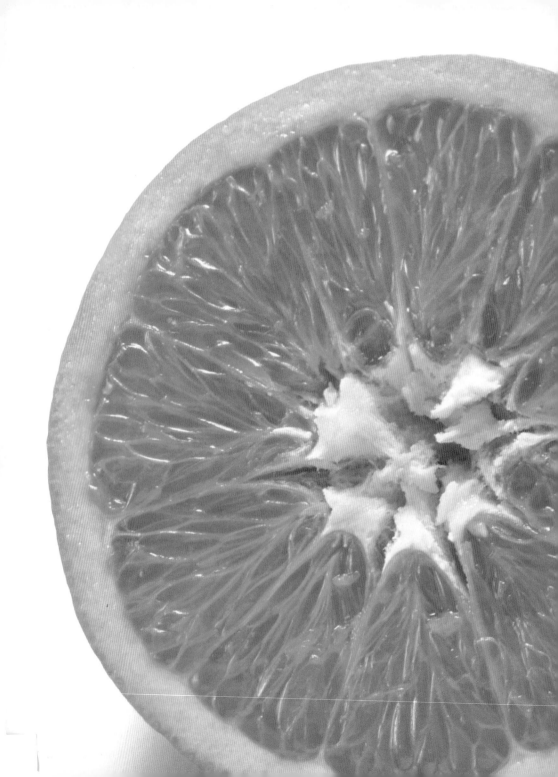

Soft Drinks and Juices

Sugar consumption is on the rise in Britain, with the average adult getting through over a pound of the white stuff per week. Much of this is "invisible" sugar – concealed in the ingredients of processed products rather than added at home. Nowhere is this more evident than in the soft drinks industry, where carbonates and concentrates have taken over and a "fruit juice" may contain as much sugar as it does fruit. Faced with these choices, water begins to look like the only healthy option.

A Spoonful of Sugar

Children in the UK eat too much sugar, and according to the Food Standards Agency "more of it comes from fizzy drinks than any other type of food or drink". These products are increasingly replacing other sources of fluid in the average diet, including tap water. This is particularly worrying because excessive consumption of high-sugar soft drinks has been linked to an increased risk of obesity and type 2 diabetes.

Campaigners in America refer to soft drinks such as coca-cola as "liquid candy", since the average glass of coke contains an astonishing seven teaspoons of sugar – or more. To put this in perspective, imagine dissolving this amount of sugar in a mug of tea or coffee. It is possible to avoid the highest sugar levels by choosing reduced-sugar "diet" drinks, although the best way to reduce your intake is to avoid consuming these products at all.

Sweeteners and Additives

Soft drinks contain very few nutrients, and are high in additives. Low sugar versions will contain an artificial sweetener such as aspartame alongside the usual colourings, flavourings and preservatives. These are useful for those on calorie-controlled diets as they do not release as much energy, and are popular with manufacturers because they are cheap to produce. Most of the major high intensity sweeteners are synthetically produced, so those who prefer natural ingredients may want to avoid them.

Colourings commonly used in soft drinks, including tartrazine (E104) and sunset yellow (E110), have been accused of causing hyperactivity and allergies in sensitive individuals. The phosphoric acid contained in most colas has been associated with bone loss that can lead to osteoporosis. However, this apparent connection may be a result of colas replacing high calcium drinks such as milk, rather than a direct effect of phosphoric acid consumption.

CAFFEINE

You would expect to find caffeine in a cup of tea or coffee, but this ingredient also appears in many of the leading soft drink brands. A can of cola may have up to 40mg of caffeine per can, compared to a cup of tea at 50mg. The presence of caffeine may be linked to the hyperactivity experienced by some children after drinking these products. Decaffeinated versions of the major brands are also available.

Energy drinks are types of soft drink that function as a pick-me-up. They usually contain substances with stimulant properties such as caffeine and taurine, both of which should be consumed in moderation. In some European countries taurine is considered a medicinal compound, and brands that include it cannot be sold alongside regular soft drinks. Caffeine is popularly used to help relieve tiredness, but in large quantities it can cause sleep disruption and may lead to addiction. Concerns have been raised over the trend for combining energy drinks with alcohol, as simultaneous intake of stimulants and depressants has been linked to heart problems in the long term.

FRUIT JUICES AND JUICE DRINKS

Fruit juices are a healthy alternative to carbonated soft drinks. A glass of pure, unsweetened fruit juice contains the same vitamins as fresh fruit, and will count as one portion of your five-a-day. Be sure to choose 100 per cent juices – those labelled as "juice drinks" may be less than 20 per cent juice, and could contain almost as much sugar as a can of fizzy drink. Some may even contain vegetable oil as a thickener, to make up for the lack of juice.

Freshly squeezed juices and smoothies are also a good choice. However, the

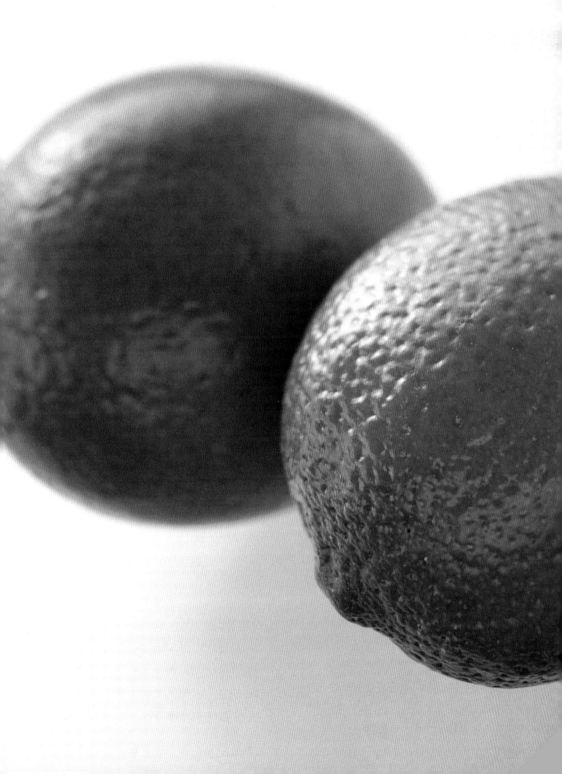

process of blending fruits for a smoothie releases sugars that can cause damage to teeth. For this reason both juices and smoothies are best drunk alongside a meal. Watch out for the salt content in some vegetable juices (such as tomato) – it can be a lot higher than you might expect.

Our Research Results

The surfeit of green in the Soft Drinks table may seem – at least at first glance – to suggest that these are healthy products, but closer inspection reveals a food category dominated by what are often referred to as "empty calories"; calories that contain few useful micronutrients and offer little in the way of nutritional value. Starting with two nutrients that are crucial for good health, protein and fibre, it is clear that these are lacking from the vast majority of the products surveyed: only Alpro Soya and Soya Light contain discernible amounts of either. Given that the majority of these products offer so few other nutrients, the fact that they are extremely low in fat, saturates and sugar is largely irrelevant.

Moreover, the one nutrient many of these drinks do contain is sugar –and lots

of it. Many of the products, including 7-up, Coca Cola and Pepsi, have more than 10g of sugar per 100g, which works out at a weighty 33g per 330ml can. Or, to put it another way, a 330ml serving of Fanta Orange contains more calories than 100g of oven chips. This may seem like a good argument for low-calorie soft drinks, but products such as Diet Coke and Pepsi Max only display straight zeros in the table because they are made with artificial additives – fewer calories, perhaps, but empty ones nonetheless.

The Good Nutrition Guide Recommends

Lowest In Sugars:
Coke Zero; Diet Coke; Pepsi Max; Red Bull; Red Bull Sugar Free

Lowest In Saturated Fats:
All products receive the top mark for saturated fat

Lowest In Salt:
All products receive the top mark for low salt

BRAND NAME	ENERGY	PROTEIN	FIBRE	CARBOHYDRATES	SUGARS	FAT	SATURATED FAT	SALT	GOOD NUTRITION GUIDE SCORE	Company group
ALPRO SOYA	43.0	3.3	0.6	2.9	2.8	1.9	0.3	0.1	100.0	Alpro
ALPRO SOYA LIGHT	21.0	2.0	1.3	0.2	0.2	1.2	0.2	0.1	100.0	Alpro
DIET TANGO	4.0	0.1	0.0	0.4	0.4	0.0	0.0	0.0	100.0	Britvic
ROBINSONS FRUIT SHOOT	5.0	0.1	0.0	0.8	0.8	0.0	0.0	0.0	100.0	Britvic
TANGO	20.0	0.1	0.0	4.4	4.4	0.0	0.0	0.0	100.0	Britvic
TANGO APPLE	18.0	0.0	0.0	4.1	4.1	0.0	0.0	0.0	100.0	Britvic
ORANGINA	42.0	0.1	0.0	10.2	1.0	0.0	0.0	0.0	100.0	Cadbury Schweppes
7-UP	46.0	0.0	0.0	11.4	11.4	0.0	0.0	0.0	87.5	Coca-Cola
COCA COLA	42.0	0.0	0.0	10.6	10.6	0.0	0.0	0.0	87.5	Coca-Cola
COKE ZERO	0.5	0.0	0.0	0.0	0.0	0.0	0.0	0.0	100.0	Coca-Cola
DIET COKE	0.5	0.0	0.0	0.0	0.0	0.0	0.0	0.0	100.0	Coca-Cola
DR PEPPER	42.0	0.0	0.0	10.5	10.5	0.0	0.0	0.0	87.5	Coca-Cola
FANTA ORANGE	53.0	0.0	0.0	10.6	10.6	0.0	0.0	0.0	87.5	Coca-Cola
LILT FRUIT CRUSH	20.0	0.0	0.0	4.5	4.5	0.0	0.0	0.0	100.0	Coca-Cola
SPRITE	44.0	0.0	0.0	10.6	10.6	0.0	0.0	0.0	87.5	Coca-Cola
RIBENA LIGHT	3.0	0.0	0.0	0.4	0.4	0.0	0.0	0.0	100.0	GlaxoSmithKline
RIBENA ORIGINAL	51.0	0.0	0.0	12.6	12.1	0.0	0.0	0.0	87.5	GlaxoSmithKline
LUCOZADE ENERGY ORANGE	70.0	0.0	0.0	17.2	0.0	0.0	0.0	0.0	100.0	Lucozade
LUCOZADE HYDROACTIVE	10.0	0.0	0.0	2.0	1.0	0.0	0.0	0.0	100.0	Lucozade
LUCOZADE SPORT	28.0	0.0	0.0	6.4	3.5	0.0	0.0	0.1	100.0	Lucozade
PEPSI	42.0	0.0	0.0	11.0	11.0	0.0	0.0	0.0	87.5	Pepsi
PEPSI MAX	0.3	0.1	0.0	0.0	0.0	0.0	0.0	0.0	100.0	Pepsi
RED BULL	45.0	0.0	0.0	11.3	0.0	0.0	0.0	0.0	100.0	Red Bull Energy
RED BULL SUGAR FREE	3.0	0.0	0.0	0.0	0.0	0.0	0.0	0.2	100.0	Red Bull Energy
D & G OLD JAMACIAN GINGER BEER	64.0	0.0	0.0	16.0	10.0	0.1	0.0	0.0	87.5	W T Foods

Key

TYPICAL SERVING SIZE: **330ML** (one can)
All figures are grammes per 100 grammes (expect Energy reading which = Kcal per100 grammes)
Source: The Ethical Company Organisation / The Good Nutrition Guide 2006 - 2008
For explantion of Good Nutrition Guide Score see the "Using the Research Tables" section

THE GOOD NUTRITION GUIDE
BEST CHOICE:
Many products with score of 100

THE GOOD NUTRITION GUIDE
WORST CHOICE:
Many products with score of 87.5

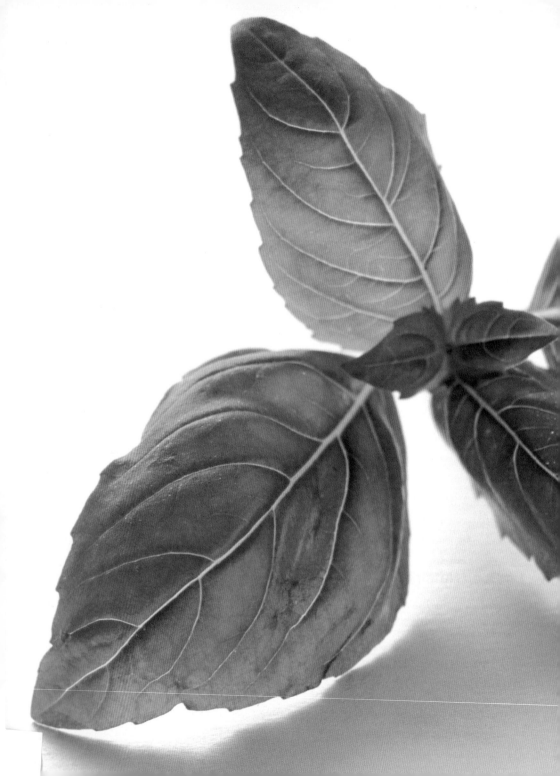

Soup

On a winter's day, there's nothing more warming than a hearty bowl of soup with a big chunk of crusty bread. The nutritional value of the meal will be determined partly by what type of soup you choose, and partly by whether it comes from a packet, a can or the chiller cabinet. As with most foods, the less processed options are nearly always better, as they contain more fibre, more fresh vegetables and fewer additives. Watch out for high salt levels and added vegetable oils.

HOW MANY VEGETABLES?

When the government's plans for a five-a-day fruit and vegetable scheme were first announced, many soup manufacturers rushed to promote their products' contribution to the daily quota. Some of these companies soon fell foul of the regulators when it emerged that their soups were also high in fat, salt and sugar. The Advertising Standards Authority upheld complaints against Knorr (who claimed that their Vie carton soups counted as three portions of vegetables) because a single serving contained 5g of salt – almost an entire day's recommended intake. Other companies were criticised for stating that their products contained more than one serving when the overall vegetable content was relatively low.

Strict labelling regulations were brought in when the scheme was officially launched in 2003, but there is still some confusion over which processed foods can contribute to our five-a-day. Look for the official five-a-day "Just Eat More (fruit and veg)" logo, which shows a series of squares coloured in according to how many portions are in the product. To apply to use this logo, manufacturers must ensure that their foods meet certain criteria – including being low in fat, sugar and salt. By late 2005, over 700 different brands were using the logo.

FINDING A HEALTHIER SOUP

For canned soups that don't carry the

five-a-day logo, look out for the following things:

High salt. Anything over 1.25g salt (0.5g sodium) per 100g is classified as "high" according to the FSA's guidelines. Remember that while most consumers would consider a can of soup to be one portion, many companies define a portion as only half a can, so you could be consuming much more salt than it might appear on the label.

Added sugar. Even savoury products such as soup may contain sweeteners. Look out for dextrose and glucose syrup, both of which are types of sugar.

High fat. While home-made soup is made with stock or water, the distinctive texture of canned soups is often created by adding vegetable oil to the liquid base. This means that even an apparently healthy option such as tomato soup may actually be high in fat. "Cream of" or "creamy" soups will usually contain more saturated fat as a result of the added cream.

Key ingredients. The ingredients list is a good indicator of the nutritional value of a can of soup. Sometimes the named ingredients – such as the vegetables in a vegetable broth – appear in very small

quantities. For example, a 400g can of Heinz Cream of Chicken Soup contains just 3 per cent chicken.

Additives. Many soups contain monosodium glutamate (E621), a flavour enhancer more readily associated with snack foods such as crisps. If the packaging lists "flavourings", this means that the product will contain one or more of the 4,000 flavourings licensed for use in the UK – but there is no way to know which one.

CANNED OR PACKET?

Although many types of processed soup have been criticised for their salt levels, packet soups are by far the worst. These powdered products typically contain potato starches and flavourings, as well as salt and sweeteners. The percentage of dried vegetables or other prominent ingredients may be very low, and they tend to contain smaller amounts of protein and fibre than the canned equivalent. In comparison, fresh or refrigerated soups are less likely to have been made with vegetable oil, and usually contain a higher proportion of meat or vegetables than both canned and packet products.

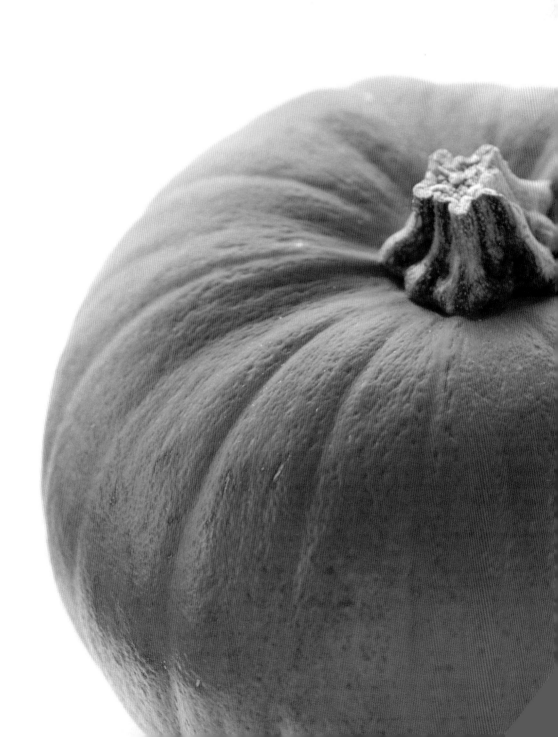

OUR RESEARCH RESULTS

Comparisons between the packet soup brands are complicated by the manufacturers' differing labelling decisions; some use figures per 100g as served, and some per 100g of powder. Within the former, there seem to be few major differences amongst the brands. Regardless of flavour, the packet soups in the Ainsley Harriott and Batchelors Cup-A-Soup ranges all contain low levels of sugars, fats and saturates and moderate amounts of salt. Like for like, the Ainsley Harriott soups are not significantly lower in calories than their competitors, despite the "lowcal" title. In the latter group there is much more variety, with many products receiving three red ratings, while others – including Knorr's Chicken Noodle Soup – have only one.

Amongst the canned soups, there is a spread of amber and green ratings, with a few products – such as Baxters Chef Selection Wild Mushroom & Smoked Bacon and New Covent Garden Chicken – displaying notably higher figures for fat and saturates. The salt figures are moderate across the board, although Spinnaker Classic Foods Seafood Gumbo comes out highest at 1.4g per 100g.

THE GOOD NUTRITION GUIDE RECOMMENDS

CANNED SOUP:

LOWEST IN SUGARS:
Lloyd Grossman Chicken & Vegetable

LOWEST IN SATURATED FATS:
Weightwatchers (all brands); Heinz Lentil Soup; Heinz Autumn Vegetable & Lentil Soup; Baxters Healthy Helpings Chunky Country Vegetable; Baxters Healthy Choice Tomato & Brown Lentil; Baxters Healthy Choice Lentil & Vegetable; Baxters Healthy Choice Italian Bean Pasta

LOWEST IN SALT:
New Covent Garden Asparagus

THE GOOD NUTRITION GUIDE BEST CHOICE:
Many products with 87.5 points

THE GOOD NUTRITION GUIDE
WORST CHOICE:

Baxters Chef Selection Carrot, Chile, Mascarpone; Baxters Chef Selection Wild Mushroom & Smoked Bacon; Baxters Luxury Broccoli, Stilton & Bacon; Baxters Luxury Cream Of Asparagus; Baxters Luxury Cullen Skink; Baxters Soup Choices Aromatic Chicken With Thai Herbs; New Covent Garden Chicken

Brand Name	Energy	Protein	Fibre	Carbohydrates	Sugars	Fat	Saturated Fat	Salt	Good Nutrition Guide Score	Company group
Amy's Low Fat Blackbean Veg	55.0	2.4	2.0	10.0	2.4	0.6	0.1	0.5	87.5	Amy's Kitchen
Amy's Low Fat Lentil	63.0	2.8	2.4	9.4	2.0	1.6	0.2	0.8	87.5	Amy's Kitchen
Amy's Low Fat Chunky Tomato	50.0	0.8	0.8	8.5	5.7	1.4	0.8	0.8	75.0	Amy's Kitchen
Smoked Bacon & Three Bean	47.0	2.4	1.7	8.4	2.4	0.4	0.1	0.5	87.5	Baxters Food Group
Baxters Chicken & Vegetable Casserole Soup	49.0	2.4	1.1	8.3	2.5	0.7	0.2	0.5	87.5	Baxters Food Group
Baxters Chef Selection Carrot, Chile, Mascarpone	53.0	1.1	0.9	4.6	3.8	3.3	2.1	0.7	62.5	Baxters Food Group
Baxters Chef Selection Red Lentil & Pancetta	68.0	3.9	0.8	8.9	2.0	1.9	0.8	0.6	87.5	Baxters Food Group
Baxters Chef Selection Wild Mushroom & Smoked Bacon	82.0	1.1	0.2	5.4	0.9	6.2	2.4	0.6	62.5	Baxters Food Group
Baxters Chilli Beef & Bean	55.0	3.7	1.8	8.5	2.2	0.7	0.3	0.5	87.5	Baxters Food Group
Baxters Favourite Chicken Broth	31.0	1.4	0.6	5.6	1.3	0.3	0.1	0.6	87.5	Baxters Food Group
Baxters Favourite Cream Of Tomato	62.0	1.0	0.3	8.4	4.9	2.7	1.1	0.5	87.5	Baxters Food Group
Baxters Favourite Highlanders Broth	47.0	1.8	0.6	6.5	0.9	1.5	0.7	0.6	87.5	Baxters Food Group
Baxters Favourite Oxtail	45.0	1.9	0.5	6.4	1.4	1.3	0.3	0.6	87.5	Baxters Food Group
Baxters Favourite Scotch Broth	46.0	1.6	0.7	6.4	1.2	0.9	0.4	0.6	87.5	Baxters Food Group
Baxters Healthy Choice Chicken & Vegetable	37.0	1.6	1.4	6.5	1.7	0.5	0.1	0.6	87.5	Baxters Food Group
Baxters Healthy Choice Italian Bean Pasta	41.0	1.7	1.3	8.2	1.4	0.2	0.0	0.6	87.5	Baxters Food Group
Baxters Healthy Choice Lentil & Vegetable	41.0	21.0	1.1	7.4	2.1	0.3	0.0	0.7	87.5	Baxters Food Group
Baxters Healthy Choice Spicy Tomato With Rice & Sweetcorn	43.0	1.3	0.6	8.7	2.0	0.3	0.1	0.5	87.5	Baxters Food Group
Baxters Healthy Choice Tomato & Brown Lentil	54.0	3.1	1.5	9.6	1.9	0.3	0.0	0.6	87.5	Baxters Food Group
Baxters Healthy Choice Vegetarian Italian Tomato With Basil	48.0	2.1	0.8	7.9	3.3	0.9	0.2	0.7	87.5	Baxters Food Group
Baxters Healthy Helpings Chunky Country Vegetable	46.0	1.9	1.5	8.9	2.6	0.3	0.0	0.6	87.5	Baxters Food Group
Baxters Luxury Broccoli, Stilton & Bacon	75.0	2.5	0.5	5.4	1.7	4.8	1.6	0.6	62.5	Baxters Food Group
Baxters Luxury Cream Of Asparagus	65.0	1.1	0.2	5.8	1.6	4.2	2.6	0.7	62.5	Baxters Food Group
Baxters Luxury Cullen Skink	85.0	5.7	0.4	7.7	3.2	3.5	2.1	0.9	62.5	Baxters Food Group
Baxters Luxury Lobster Bisque	44.0	2.7	0.1	3.8	1.6	2.0	1.2	0.7	87.5	Baxters Food Group
Baxters Luxury Mushroom Pottage	78.0	1.5	0.3	6.6	2.1	5.1	1.2	0.8	75.0	Baxters Food Group
Baxters Pumpkin Sweetcorn & Hot Sweet Chilli	49.0	1.2	1.0	9.8	3.0	0.6	0.2	0.6	87.5	Baxters Food Group
Baxters Soup Choices Aromatic Chicken With Thai Herbs	67.0	1.8	0.3	5.7	1.9	4.3	2.4	0.6	62.5	Baxters Food Group
Baxters Soup Choices Carrot Crème Fraiche & Coriander	46.0	0.8	0.9	6.2	3.2	2.0	1.0	0.7	87.5	Baxters Food Group
Baxters Soup Choices Tomato & Herbs	51.0	1.1	0.7	7.0	4.3	2.1	1.0	0.7	87.5	Baxters Food Group
Baxters Vegetable Country Garden Soup	33.0	1.0	0.8	6.0	1.4	0.5	0.3	0.5	87.5	Baxters Food Group
Grossman Carrot & Coriander Soup	51.0	0.6	1.0	6.4	3.7	2.5	0.7	0.5	87.5	Chivers Hartley
Grossman Chicken & Vegetable	68.0	0.5	0.6	8.0	0.2	3.8	1.1	0.7	75.0	Chivers Hartley
Spinnaker Classic Bouillabaisse	92.0	4.2	0.5	6.3	2.0	5.4	1.0	1.0	75.0	Danfoods
Spinnaker Classic Foods Seafood Gumbo	83.0	4.5	0.5	5.1	0.5	4.8	1.0	1.4	75.0	Danfoods

Key

Typical serving size: 200ml (half a standard can)

All figures are grammes per 100 grammes (expect Energy reading which = Kcal per100 grammes)

Source: The Ethical Company Organisation / The Good Nutrition Guide 2006 - 2008

For explantion of Good Nutrition Guide Score see the "Using the Research Tables" section

BRAND NAME	ENERGY	PROTEIN	FIBRE	CARBOHYDRATES	SUGARS	FAT	SATURATED FAT	SALT	GOOD NUTRITION GUIDE SCORE	Company group
HAWKWARD FOODS TUSCAN BEAN SOUP	43.0	2.6	2.0	6.3	1.3	0.8	0.1	0.8	87.5	Hawkward Foods
HAWKWARD ORGANIC BARLEY BROTH	25.0	1.4	0.9	3.9	1.2	0.4	0.1	0.8	87.5	Hawkward Foods
HAWKWARD ORGANIC LEEK & POTATO SOUP	48.0	1.7	0.9	7.4	0.8	1.3	0.2	0.7	87.5	Hawkward Foods
HEINZ AUTUMN VEGETABLE & LENTIL SOUP	46.0	2.3	1.0	8.6	1.5	0.3	0.0	0.6	87.5	Heinz
HEINZ BIG SOUP CHICKEN & VEGETABLE	47.0	2.9	0.9	7.4	1.6	0.6	0.2	0.7	87.5	Heinz
HEINZ CHICKEN NOODLE SOUP	27.0	1.1	0.2	5.1	1.1	0.3	0.1	0.7	87.5	Heinz
HEINZ CREAM OF MUSHROOM	52.0	1.6	0.1	5.2	2.1	2.8	0.4	0.7	87.5	Heinz
HEINZ CREAM OF TOMATO	57.0	0.9	0.4	6.6	4.9	3.0	0.2	0.7	87.5	Heinz
HEINZ CREAM OF TOMATO WITH A HINT OF BASIL	56.0	0.9	0.4	6.7	4.9	2.9	0.2	0.7	87.5	Heinz
HEINZ GARDEN PEA & HAM SOUP	44.0	2.4	1.2	5.9	0.9	1.2	0.2	0.7	87.5	Heinz
HEINZ LENTIL SOUP	43.0	2.3	1.0	3.0	0.9	0.2	0.0	0.6	87.5	Heinz
HEINZ MINESTRONE	42.0	1.0	0.8	5.8	1.7	1.6	0.2	0.7	87.5	Heinz
HEINZ MUG SIZE CREAM OF CHICKEN	49.0	1.5	0.1	4.5	1.1	2.7	0.4	0.6	87.5	Heinz
HEINZ MUG SIZE VEGETABLE SOUP	43.0	1.0	0.9	8.2	3.2	0.7	0.1	0.7	87.5	Heinz
HEINZ MULLIGATAWNY BEEF CURRY SOUP	54.0	2.0	0.6	7.2	3.4	1.9	0.3	0.7	87.5	Heinz
HEINZ MUSHROOM POTTAGE	59.0	0.9	0.1	5.5	0.9	3.8	0.7	0.7	75.0	Heinz
HEINZ ORGANIC TOMATO	55.0	1.0	0.4	7.0	4.9	2.6	0.9	0.7	87.5	Heinz
HEINZ OXTAIL	39.0	1.9	0.3	6.7	1.9	0.5	0.2	0.6	87.5	Heinz
HEINZ POTATO & LEEK	4.6	0.8	0.6	6.7	0.8	1.8	1.1	0.7	87.5	Heinz
HEINZ SCOTCH BROTH	35.0	12.0	0.6	5.8	0.8	0.7	0.3	0.7	87.5	Heinz
HEINZ SPECIAL ROAST VEGETABLE & BARLEY BROTH	47.0	0.9	1.1	7.4	1.7	1.5	0.1	0.7	87.5	Heinz
HEINZ SPECIAL, CREAMY ROASTED CHICKEN WITH ROSEMARY	58.0	2.5	0.2	5.7	0.5	2.8	1.5	0.7	87.5	Heinz
WEIGHTWATCHERS CARROT & LENTIL	29.0	1.3	0.7	5.7	1.6	0.1	0.0	0.7	87.5	Heinz
WEIGHTWATCHERS COUNTRY VEGETABLE SOUP	31.0	1.1	1.0	6.1	1.0	0.2	0.0	0.6	87.5	Heinz
WEIGHTWATCHERS TOMATO SOUP	25.0	0.7	0.3	4.5	2.7	0.5	0.0	0.6	87.5	Heinz
NEW COVENT GARDEN ASPARAGUS	37.0	0.9	0.9	4.5	1.0	1.7	1.0	0.4	87.5	New Covent Garden Company
NEW COVENT GARDEN CARROT & CORIANDER	40.0	0.8	0.5	6.2	2.8	1.3	0.8	0.6	87.5	New Covent Garden Company
NEW COVENT GARDEN CHICKEN	85.0	3.8	0.6	5.4	1.0	5.4	2.4	0.6	62.5	New Covent Garden Company
NEW COVENT GARDEN LEEK & POTATO	42.0	0.6	0.8	7.0	1.2	1.3	0.8	0.6	87.5	New Covent Garden Company
NEW COVENT GARDEN WILD MUSHROOM	52.0	0.9	0.7	7.4	0.6	2.1	1.3	0.7	87.5	New Covent Garden Company
NEW COVENT GARDEN WINTER VEGETABLES	59.0	3.4	1.6	6.1	2.6	2.3	1.3	0.5	87.5	New Covent Garden Company
SEEDS OF CHANGE ORGANIC CARROT & CORIANDER	37.0	0.6	1.1	4.7	1.6	1.8	1.1	1.1	87.5	Seeds Of Change
SEEDS OF CHANGE ORGANIC CREAMY TOMATO	64.0	1.2	0.5	11.0	5.9	1.7	1.3	1.1	75.0	Seeds Of Change
SEEDS OF CHANGE ORGANIC MINESTRONE	64.0	1.4	1.4	7.1	2.5	3.3	0.5	0.9	75.0	Seeds Of Change
SEEDS OF CHANGE ORGANIC SPICY LENTIL	70.0	2.8	1.2	9.6	2.6	2.2	0.3	1.1	87.5	Seeds Of Change
SEEDS OF CHANGE ORGANIC THREE BEAN SOUP	55.0	1.1	1.7	9.0	2.5	1.3	0.2	1.0	87.5	Seeds Of Change

Key

TYPICAL SERVING SIZE: 200ML (half a standard can)

All figures are grammes per 100 grammes (expect Energy reading which = Kcal per100 grammes)

Source: The Ethical Company Organisation / The Good Nutrition Guide 2006 - 2008

For explantion of Good Nutrition Guide Score see the "Using the Research Tables" section

PACKET SOUP:

LOWEST IN SUGARS:

Ainsley Harriott's Low Cal Hi Taste Leek, Potato & Pea Cup Soup

LOWEST IN SATURATED FATS:

Ainsley Harriott's Hot & Sour Cup Soup; Ainsley Harriott's Low Cal Hi Taste Spicy Lentil Cup Soup; Ainsley Harriott's Scottish Style Chicken & Leek Soup

LOWEST IN SALT:

Ainsley Harriott's Low Cal Hi Taste Asparagus Cup Soup; Ainsley Harriott's Lowcal Hi Taste Vegetable Cup Soup

THE GOOD NUTRITION GUIDE BEST CHOICE:

Ainsley Harriott's Low Cal Hi Taste Asparagus Cup Soup; Ainsley Harriott's Lowcal Hi Taste Vegetable Cup Soup

THE GOOD NUTRITION GUIDE WORST CHOICE:

Of the products labelled per 100g as served: many on 87.5 points

Of the products labelled per 100g of powder: Symingtons Tomato & Basil; Knorr Asparagus Soup; Knorr Carrot & Coriander Soup; Knorr Golden Vegetable Soup; Knorr Soups Of The World English Broccoli & Stilton

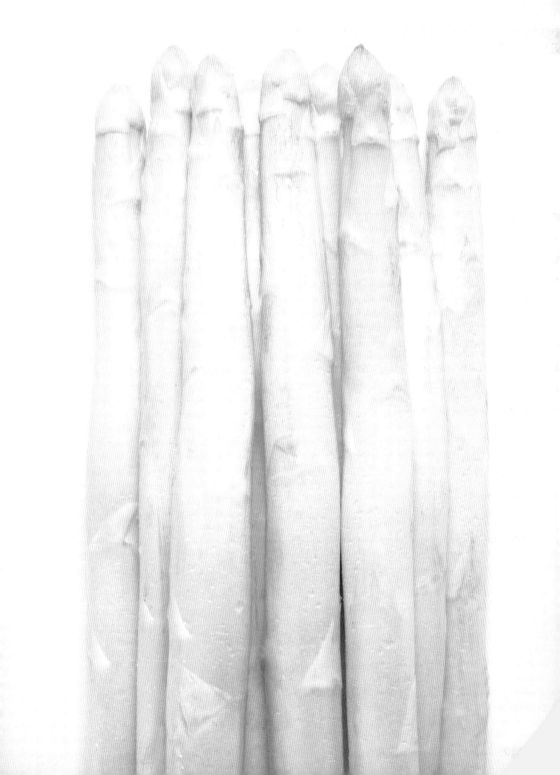

BRAND NAME	ENERGY	PROTEIN	FIBRE	CARBOHYDRATES	SUGARS	FAT	SATURATED FAT	SALT	GOOD NUTRITION GUIDE SCORE	Company group
Ainsley Harriott's Hot & Sour Cup Soup	24.0	0.5	1.0	5.4	1.1	0.0	0.0	1.0	87.5	Brand Partnerships
Ainsley Harriott's Low Cal Hi Taste Asparagus Cup Soup	36.0	0.5	0.5	6.4	0.7	0.9	0.5	0.3	100.0	Brand Partnerships
Ainsley Harriott's Low Cal Hi Taste Leek, Potato & Pea Cup Soup	33.0	1.2	0.4	6.3	0.3	0.3	0.2	0.5	87.5	Brand Partnerships
Ainsley Harriott's Low Cal Hi Taste Spicy Lentil Cup Soup	30.0	1.2	0.5	6.0	0.9	0.1	0.0	0.5	87.5	Brand Partnerships
Ainsley Harriott's Lowcal Hi Taste Vegetable Cup Soup	34.0	0.9	0.4	6.8	1.1	0.3	0.2	0.3	100.0	Brand Partnerships
Ainsley Harriott's New England Style Vegetable Chowder Cup Soup	36.0	0.6	1.2	5.8	0.9	1.2	0.4	1.0	87.5	Brand Partnerships
Ainsley Harriott's Scottish Style Chicken & Leek Soup	28.0	0.5	0.8	6.1	2.5	0.2	0.0	0.8	87.5	Brand Partnerships
Ainsley Harriott's Wonderfully Wild Mushroom Cup Soup	38.0	0.4	0.8	5.5	0.6	1.6	1.0	1.3	87.5	Brand Partnerships
Batchelors Cup-A-Soup Chicken & Vegetable	52.0	0.5	0.8	6.9	1.2	2.5	1.3	0.9	87.5	Campbell Grocery Products
Batchelors Cup-A-Soup Cream of Mushroom	47.0	0.3	0.8	5.9	0.9	2.5	1.2	0.7	87.5	Campbell Grocery Products
Batchelors Cup-A-Soup Creamy Broccoli & Cauliflower	42.0	0.6	1.1	5.3	1.3	2.0	1.0	0.9	87.5	Campbell Grocery Products
Batchelors Cup-A-Soup Oxtail	33.0	0.9	0.3	4.4	0.8	1.3	0.6	1.1	87.5	Campbell Grocery Products
Batchelors Cup-A-Soup Tomato	36.0	0.3	0.3	6.7	3.7	0.9	0.4	1.2	87.5	Campbell Grocery Products
Batchelors Minestrone Cup-A-Soup	38.0	0.6	0.5	6.4	2.0	1.1	0.5	0.9	87.5	Campbell Grocery Products
Batchelor's Cup-A-Soup Chicken	33.0	0.4	0.6	3.3	0.9	2.0	1.0	0.9	87.5	Campbell Grocery Products
Batchelor's Cup-A-Soup Golden Vegetable	33.0	0.4	0.4	5.7	1.3	0.9	0.4	1.0	87.5	Campbell Grocery Products
Batchelor's Slim-A-Soup Cajun Spicy Vegetable	25.0	0.8	0.8	4.5	2.7	0.4	0.2	1.0	87.5	HL Foods
Batchelor's Slim-A-Soup Chicken Noodle & Vegetable	27.0	0.8	0.6	4.9	1.2	0.5	0.2	0.7	87.5	HL Foods
Batchelor's Slim-A-Soup Minestrone & Croutons	27.0	0.6	0.6	4.9	1.9	0.5	0.2	1.1	87.5	HL Foods

Key

TYPICAL SERVING SIZE: 300ML (one soup sachet per person)

All figures are grammes per 100 grammes (expect Energy reading which = Kcal per100 grammes)

Source: The Ethical Company Organisation / The Good Nutrition Guide 2006 - 2008

For explantion of Good Nutrition Guide Score see the "Using the Research Tables" section

Brand Name	Energy	Protein	Fibre	Carbohydrates	Sugars	Fat	Saturated Fat	Salt	Good Nutrition Guide Score	Company group
Symingtons Chicken & Leek With Croutons	409.0	4.3	3.7	62.8	9.4	15.6	8.6	6.8	25.0	Brand Partnerships
Symingtons French Onion	335.0	5.2	8.5	70.3	10.7	3.7	1.7	7.5	37.5	Brand Partnerships
Symingtons Mulligatawny	367.0	5.3	2.9	70.5	11.8	7.1	3.6	8.8	37.5	Brand Partnerships
Symingtons Shropshire Pea	356.0	8.1	5.4	70.8	9.5	4.4	2.0	6.0	37.5	Brand Partnerships
Symingtons Tomato & Basil	382.0	4.6	3.3	69.1	29.7	9.7	5.5	5.0	12.5	Brand Partnerships
Knorr Asparagus Soup	455.0	6.3	2.1	47.9	6.4	26.4	16.7	4.2	12.5	Unilever
Knorr Carrot & Coriander Soup	378.0	7.7	10.3	47.2	22.6	17.2	10.4	3.6	12.5	Unilever
Knorr Chicken Noodle Soup	328.0	14.9	3.5	56.7	2.0	4.6	0.2	4.9	62.5	Unilever
Knorr Florida Spring Vegetable Soup	277.0	10.0	10.4	43.3	8.9	6.8	3.5	6.8	37.5	Unilever
Knorr Golden Vegetable Soup	409.0	10.0	4.6	47.8	16.7	19.5	12.2	4.0	12.5	Unilever
Knorr Leek & Chicken Soup	440.0	10.6	1.6	36.0	4.2	28.1	16.1	4.6	25.0	Unilever
Knorr Soups Of The World Austrian Cream Of Herb Soup	505.0	7.6	2.3	41.2	4.1	34.3	23.8	2.8	25.0	Unilever
Knorr Soups Of The World English Broccoli & Stilton	519.0	11.2	3.6	30.8	7.5	39.0	23.9	3.6	12.5	Unilever
Knorr Soups Of The World French Onion Soup	317.0	11.5	10.3	52.3	21.1	6.3	3.2	3.0	25.0	Unilever
Knorr Thick Vegetable Soup	353.0	10.2	5.9	54.7	8.5	10.2	6.3	4.6	25.0	Unilever

Key

Typical serving size: 300ml (one soup sachet serves 3-4 people)

All figures are grammes per 100 grammes (expect Energy reading which = Kcal per100 grammes)

Source: The Ethical Company Organisation / The Good Nutrition Guide 2006 - 2008

For explantion of Good Nutrition Guide Score see the "Using the Research Tables" section

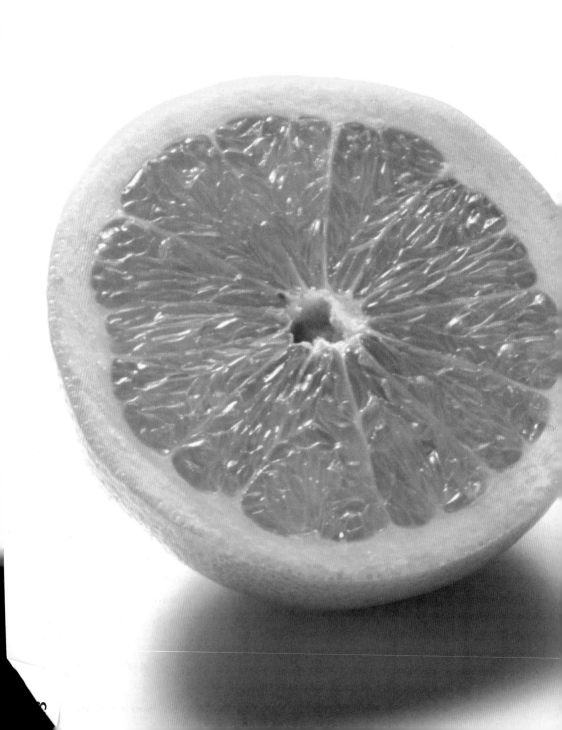

Sweets

Although there's nothing wrong with a few sweets every now and then, some companies would like us to believe that their products aren't just occasional sugary treats but have actual nutritional value. Claims that fruit chews and boiled sweets can contribute to our recommended daily intake of vitamin C indicate the extent to which simple nutritional advice has been obfuscated by the food industry's marketing tactics. Trust your instincts: if it's in the confectionery section, it's probably high in sugar and low in the nutrients that are important to a balanced diet.

MARKETING

Today's children consume 25 times more confectionery than children 50 years ago. This could be down to a wide range of factors, including increased availability of sweets in school tuck shops and vending machines, children having more pocket money to spend and more effective marketing from manufacturers. Companies are developing increasingly shrewd campaigns to promote their products to children. Many of these involve the internet, where advertising methods and nutritional claims are less tightly policed than they are on television and in print.

One of the more brazen marketing techniques is the health claim. We all know that too many sweets are bad for us, but this doesn't stop companies from using nutritional claims to market their high sugar confectionary. Some of these are aimed at adults, but others – more worryingly – appear on websites that also appeal to children. The website for Chupa Chups lollies, for example, makes many claims, amongst them being that "the act of sucking stimulates saliva and increases the flow of oxygen. This is beneficial both for growth and the immune functions, [and] helps improve your body's natural defenses against many common illnesses". They also state: "50 per cent of ex-smokers point out that Chupa Chups lollipops help [them] to stop smoking or to smoke less".

Vitamin C

Many companies use added vitamin C as a selling point for their sweets. According to Fox's website, a serving of six Glacier Fruits provides you with 40 per cent of the recommended daily allowance of vitamin C. The makers of Starburst claim on their website that the chewy sweets are "high in vitamin C", while many other sweet products use the phrase "made with real fruit juice". All of these sweets are extremely high in sugar, which makes any positive nutrition claims potentially misleading. Confectionery is no substitute for a diet rich in fresh fruit and vegetables, which will provide more than enough vitamin C, as well as fibre and other important vitamins and minerals that aren't found in confectionary.

Added Ingredients

The main ingredient in sweets and mints is sugar, which may appear in many different forms. Glucose syrup is often used as a basis for gummy sweets and chews, while sweeteners such as aspartame, sorbitol and sucralose appear in many mints and gums. In most cases, the sugar content will be reflected in the high proportion of "carbohydrates (of which sugars)" on the nutrition label. Dental association logos such as the "Tooth White" and "Tooth Friendly" symbols show that a product has been approved because it does not promote the development of cavities. Sugar free sweets and lollies usually contain a substitute sweetener such as xylitol. This is a natural sweetener and has the E number 967.

Hydrogenated vegetable oil is surprisingly common in sweets, so if you want to avoid trans fats look out for it on the label. Many confectionary products use pork gelatine, so will not be suitable for vegetarians. Food colourings are used in most sweets and novelty confectionary. Some artificial colourings, particularly tartrazine (E102) and quinoline yellow (E104), have been anecdotally linked to hyperactivity in children. Products that claim they contain "no artificial colours" will use colourings from natural sources, such as curcumin (E100), which is made from turmeric root.

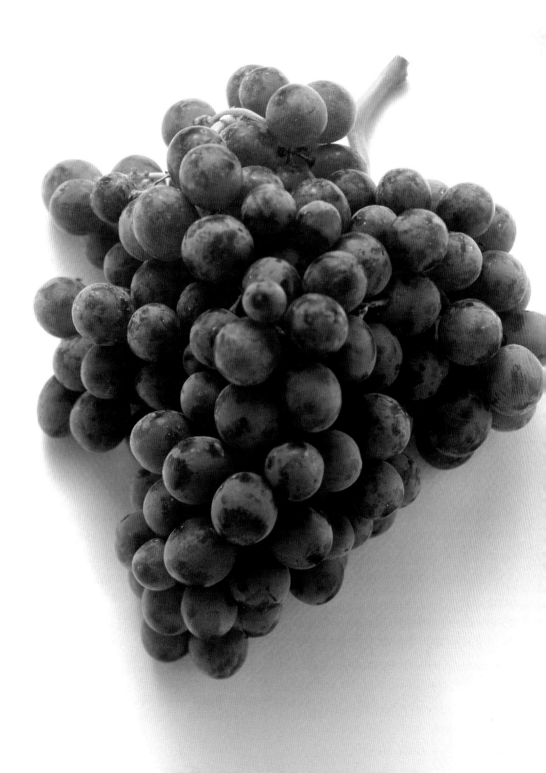

Our Research Results

The three highest sugar products in the table are all mints: Bassetts Mint Imperials at 98.1g per 100g, Polo at 95.8g and Trebor Extra Strong Peppermint at 95g. Lowest in sugar are Liquorice Catherine Wheels at 43.3g per 100g, which is still more than enough to get them a "high" rating. Like the soft drinks research, the Sweets table displays a familiar discrepancy between good ratings and good nutrition. Many of these sugary products have a reasonable score overall – precisely because they contain very little apart from sugar. Many are low in fat, saturates and salt, and contain only a trace of other nutrients: there is no protein or fibre in Trebor Soft Mints, Skittles, Starbust and many others. Those who expect Skittles and Starburst to be made almost entirely from sugar may be surprised to discover that they receive an amber rating for fats and saturates.

They are not the only sweets in the table to be higher in fat. At the top of the list, Peanut M&Ms contain 26.8g fat and 11g saturates, and are also the highest in calories overall. Nut-free but not far behind, Smarties boast 16.7g fat and 10.8g saturates, and Cadbury Chocolate Eclairs contain a similar 10.1g saturates. Storck's creamy Werther's Originals are also a source of saturates, with 6.1g per 100g. Sodium is a potential concern even in this sugary product category, where four products receive an amber rating for salt. Two of these, Haribo Liquorice Pontefract Cakes and Werther's Original, have 1g or more of salt. Cadbury Chocolate Eclairs and Maynard Wine Gums are the only other products to contain more than 0.3g of salt.

The Good Nutrition Guide Recommends

Lowest In Sugars:
Liquorice Catherine Wheels

Lowest In Saturated Fats:
Bassetts Jelly Babies; Trebor Extra Strong Peppermint; Trebor Soft Mints Peppermint; Haribo Kiddies Supermix; Rowntrees Fruit Gums; Rowntrees Fruit Pastilles

Brand Name	Energy	Protein	Fibre	Carbohydrates	Sugars	Fat	Saturated Fat	Salt	Good Nutrition Guide Score	Company group
Bassetts Dessert Allsorts	375.0	1.9	0.3	86.9	67.3	2.1	1.2	0.0	75.0	Cadbury Schweppes
Bassetts Jelly Babies	335.0	3.6	0.0	80.0	75.7	0.0	0.0	0.0	75.0	Cadbury Schweppes
Bassetts Mint Imperials	400.0	0.4	0.0	98.1	98.1	0.5	0.5	0.0	75.0	Cadbury Schweppes
Chocolate Eclairs	455.0	4.5	0.1	68.8	46.4	17.9	10.1	0.8	25.0	Cadbury Schweppes
Maynards Wine Gums	325.0	5.8	0.0	74.2	55.6	0.6	0.5	0.5	62.5	Cadbury Schweppes
Trebor Extra Strong Peppermint	395.0	0.3	0.0	98.7	95.0	0.0	0.0	0.0	75.0	Cadbury Schweppes
Trebor Soft Mints Peppermint	355.0	0.0	0.0	88.9	70.1	0.0	0.0	0.1	75.0	Cadbury Schweppes
Haribo Kiddies Supermix	344.0	6.6	0.3	79.0	63.4	0.2	0.1	0.0	75.0	Dunhills
Haribo Liquorice Pontefract Cakes	296.0	5.3	5.6	68.2	46.6	0.2	0.1	1.3	62.5	Dunhills
Haribo Star Mix	344.0	6.6	0.3	79.0	63.4	0.2	0.1	0.0	75.0	Dunhills
Chewits	378.0	0.3	0.0	86.9	53.9	2.7	1.8	0.3	62.5	Leaf
Peanut M&M's	516.0	9.8	2.8	59.0	52.4	26.8	11.0	0.1	25.0	Masterfoods
Skittles	404.0	0.0	0.0	91.5	76.4	4.2	1.7	0.0	50.0	Masterfoods
Starburst	404.0	0.0	0.0	83.5	61.1	7.4	4.0	0.0	50.0	Masterfoods
Barrat's Nougat	365.0	4.3	0.9	79.5	56.0	3.5	2.0	0.3	50.0	Monkhill Confectionary
Liquorice Catherine Wheels	290.0	3.8	0.7	67.2	43.3	0.3	0.1	0.3	75.0	Monkhill Confectionary
Polo	402.0	0.0	0.0	98.2	95.8	1.0	1.0	0.0	75.0	Nestle
Rowntrees Fruit Gums	334.0	4.8	0.0	81.3	44.0	0.2	0.0	0.3	75.0	Nestle
Rowntrees Fruit Pastilles	350.0	4.3	0.0	83.4	57.1	0.0	0.0	0.1	75.0	Nestle
Smarties	461.0	4.0	0.6	73.6	68.3	16.7	10.8	0.1	37.5	Nestle
Werther's Original	424.0	0.1	0.1	85.7	70.2	8.9	6.1	1.0	25.0	Storck

Key

Typical serving size: 50g (one pack)
All figures are grammes per 100 grammes (expect Energy reading which = Kcal per100 grammes)
Source: The Ethical Company Organisation / The Good Nutrition Guide 2006 - 2008
For explantion of Good Nutrition Guide Score see the "Using the Research Tables" section

Lowest In Salt:
Bassetts Dessert Allsorts; Bassetts Jelly Babies; Bassetts Mint Imperials; Trebor Extra Strong Peppermint; Haribo Kiddies Supermix; Haribo Star Mix; Skittles; Starburst; Polo

The Good Nutrition Guide Best Choice:
Many on 75 points

The Good Nutrition Guide Worst Choice:
Chocolate Eclairs; Peanut M&M's; Werther's Original

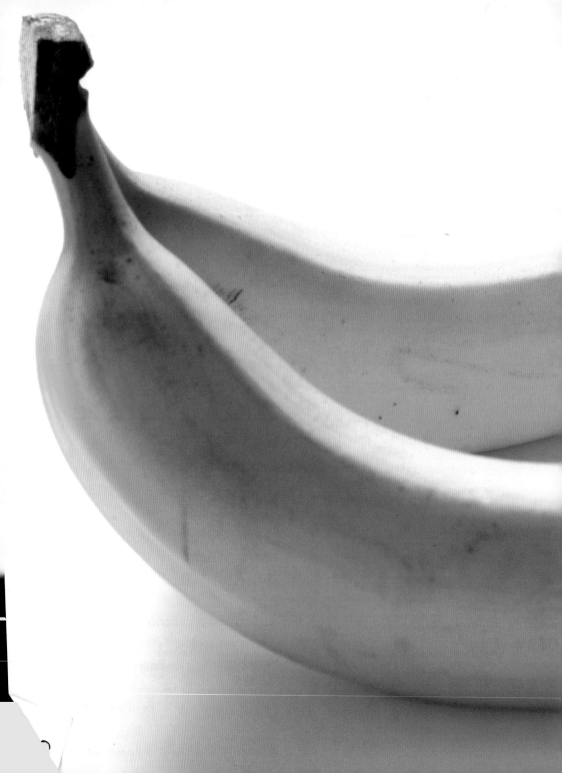

Yoghurts

As a breakfast item, a snack, an alternative to cream or a dessert in itself, yoghurt is a versatile food and a good source of protein and calcium. With natural, Greek and organic yoghurts available as well as flavoured versions from all the major brands, there are plenty of different types to choose from. Fat and sugar content are the main concerns in this product category – and watch out for yoghurts that have the "flavour" of an ingredient without actually containing it.

FLAVOUR OR FLAVOURED?

The description given on the packaging will provide a good indication as to the yoghurt's nutritional value. It may seem like a minor difference, but there is a crucial distinction between strawberry "flavour" yoghurt and strawberry "flavoured" yoghurt. While both terms would appear to suggest that the yoghurt contains real pieces of strawberry (which may contribute to your five-a-day) in fact only one of the products will have been anywhere near fresh fruit. By law, a "flavoured" product must be made with actual fruit, while one that contains fruit "flavour" will get its taste from additives – and not a piece of fruit in sight.

To help prevent confusion, there are also rules about which types of product can display pictures of their ingredients. A "strawberry flavoured" yoghurt would be allowed to carry images of real strawberries, while a "strawberry flavour" one would not. When buying flavoured yoghurt, it is still important to check exactly how much of the ingredient appears in the product. The further down the ingredients list, the less fruit it contains.

ADDITIVES

Companies are keen for us to believe that their yoghurts are full of fresh goodness, but sometimes it is just canny marketing. In July 2006, Nestlé was forced to withdraw one of its magazine adverts following criticism from the Advertising Standards Authority. The ad for Ski yoghurt used the slogan "keep it simple – no artificial colour, sweetener or preservative", when the product actually contained synthetic additives.

Most big brand yoghurts use a wide variety of additives, including colourings and sweeteners. Note that some companies make a distinction between sweeteners (meaning high intensity artificial sweeteners such as aspartame) and added sugar. So while the Müller website states that their Corner Healthy Balance yoghurts contain "no sweeteners", a look at the ingredients list reveals that their Healthy Balance Strawberry yoghurt does include plenty of added sugar – in the form of honey, sugar and fructose. Don't be fooled into thinking that a no-added-sweeteners product is a no-added-sugar product.

Try organic brands for yoghurts made with the minimum number of additives. Many use no synthetic additives at all, and simply flavour their products with cane sugar and real fruit. Natural yoghurt is a good option as it contains no added sugar, and can be combined with fresh fruit at home. Greek yoghurts are traditionally made with added cream, so although they contain no added sugar they may be high in saturated fat. Equally, yoghurts labelled with descriptive terms such as "luxury" or "indulgent" may contain cream – and could contain more calories than a refrigerated dessert.

Low Fat/Low Sugar

Yoghurts that proclaim themselves "fat-free" or "low fat" will probably be made from either semi-skimmed or skimmed milk – wholemilk products will be higher in fat and saturates. However, a phrase such as "reduced fat" refers only to one brand, so there's a chance that the standard versions of other brands will contain even lower levels of fat. Similarly, low fat does not always equate to low calorie: many use extra sugar in its place.

Similarly, there are no fixed definitions for terms such as "low sugar" or "light". This means that the product is not guaranteed to match a certain nutritional profile. Low sugar products may actually be higher in additives, as they get their sweetness from synthetic substitutes such as acesulfame K (E950). These yoghurts may also be made with fruit juice or

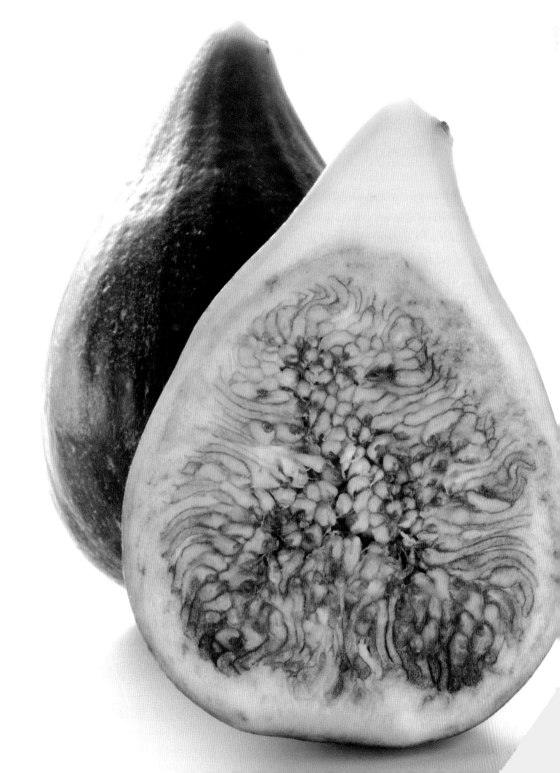

concentrate rather than fruit pieces, which will affect their nutrient content.

OUR RESEARCH RESULTS

Perhaps the most eye-catching aspect of the Yoghurts table is the unbroken line of green on the bottom row. Every single product in this category has a low rating for salt – a notable occurrence, given that even the Sweets table contains a few flashes of amber. The Benecol Classic Low Fat Bio Yoghurt and Onken Wholegrain Biopot Peach both have a resounding zero for salt. Slightly less positive, perhaps, are the figures for sugars, which suggest that many of the products may contain added sugar beyond the sugars found naturally in milk. The highest figures for sugar belong to Onken Wholegrain Biopot Peach at 14.6g per 100g and Flora Pro-activ at 14.3g. Non-flavoured products, such as Rachel's Organic Greek Style and Woodlands Park Dairy's Sheep's Milk Yoghurt, tend to be much lower in sugar.

Despite this, Rachel's Organic Greek Style is the highest in both fats and saturates in the table, and is the only product to receive a red rating for saturated fat. Many other yoghurts,

including Muller's Fruit Corner Raspberry and Nestlé's Fromage Frais Dessert, contain a moderate amount of fat; Raspberry Activia and Petit Filous both have a low fat level but moderate amounts of saturates. Of the less scrutinised nutrients, Nestlé's Fromage Frais is highest in protein overall, at 7g per 100g, closely followed by Petit Filous at 6.8g. Shape (Mango) is highest in fibre. Onken Natural Biopot contains the fewest calories, while Nestlé's Fromage Frais Desert and Rachel's Organic Greek Style yoghurt have the most at 115 and 116kcal per 100g.

THE GOOD NUTRITION GUIDE RECOMMENDS

LOWEST IN SUGARS:
Sheep's Milk Yoghurt

LOWEST IN SATURATED FATS:
Benecol Classic Low Fat Bio Yoghurt

LOWEST IN SALT:
Benecol Classic Low Fat Bio Yoghurt; Onken Wholegrain Biopot Peach

Brand Name	Energy	Protein	Fibre	Carbohydrates	Sugars	Fat	Saturated Fat	Salt	Good Nutrition Guide Score	Company group
Activia (Raspberry)	90.0	3.5	2.0	12.8	12.2	2.8	1.7	0.3	75.0	Danone
Shape (Mango)	63.0	6.6	2.2	9.0	8.7	0.1	0.1	0.2	87.5	Danone
Benecol Classic Low Fat Bio Yoghurt	78.0	3.8	0.2	14.2	12.4	0.6	0.0	0.0	87.5	McNeil Nutritionals
Fruit Corner Raspberry	107.0	3.9	1.0	14.0	13.3	3.9	2.4	0.3	62.5	Muller Dairy
Little Stars (Blackcurrent)	92.0	4.7	0.6	13.6	12.8	1.7	1.1	0.3	87.5	Muller Dairy
Muller Vitality (Blueberry)	97.0	4.8	0.7	14.0	14.0	1.9	1.2	0.3	87.5	Muller Dairy
Fromage Frais Dessert	115.0	7.0	0.1	14.1	13.8	3.4	2.1	0.1	62.5	Nestle
Onken Natural Biopot	48.0	5.4	0.0	6.4	6.3	0.1	0.1	0.1	87.5	Onken Dairy
Onken Wholegrain Biopot Peach	112.0	4.2	0.4	17.6	14.6	2.7	1.8	0.0	75.0	Onken Dairy
Little Rachel's Organic Fruit Yoghurts (Strawberry)	97.0	3.6	0.1	13.7	13.0	3.1	1.9	0.1	62.5	Rachel's Dairy
Rachel's Organic Rhubarb	83.0	4.0	0.1	13.1	13.1	1.6	1.0	0.1	87.5	Rachel's Dairy
Rachel's Organic Greek Style	116.0	3.7	0.4	5.0	5.0	9.0	5.8	0.1	62.5	Rachel's Dairy
Flora Pro-activ	78.0	3.9	0.2	14.5	14.3	0.5	0.1	0.3	87.5	Unilever
Sheep's Milk Yoghurt	92.0	5.2	0.0	4.8	4.8	5.8	3.8	0.3	75.0	Woodlands Park Dairy
Organic Live Yoghurt	82.0	4.5	0.0	6.6	6.6	4.2	2.6	0.3	62.5	Yeo Valley
Petit Filous	104.0	6.8	0.3	12.7	12.3	2.9	2.0	0.1	75.0	Yoplait

Key

Typical serving size: 150g (one pot)

All figures are grammes per 100 grammes (expect Energy reading which = Kcal per 100 grammes)

Source: The Ethical Company Organisation / The Good Nutrition Guide 2006 - 2008

For explantion of Good Nutrition Guide Score see the "Using the Research Tables" section

The Good Nutrition Guide Best Choice:

Shape (Mango); Benecol Classic Low Fat Bio Yoghurt; Little Stars (Blackcurrent); Muller Vitality (Blueberry); Onken Natural Biopot; Rachel's Organic Rhubarb; Flora Pro-activ

The Good Nutrition Guide Worst Choice:

Muller Fruit Corner Raspberry; Nestle Fromage Frais Dessert; Little Rachel's Organic Fruit Yoghurts (Strawberry); Rachel's Organic Greek Style; Yeo Valley Organic Live Yoghurt

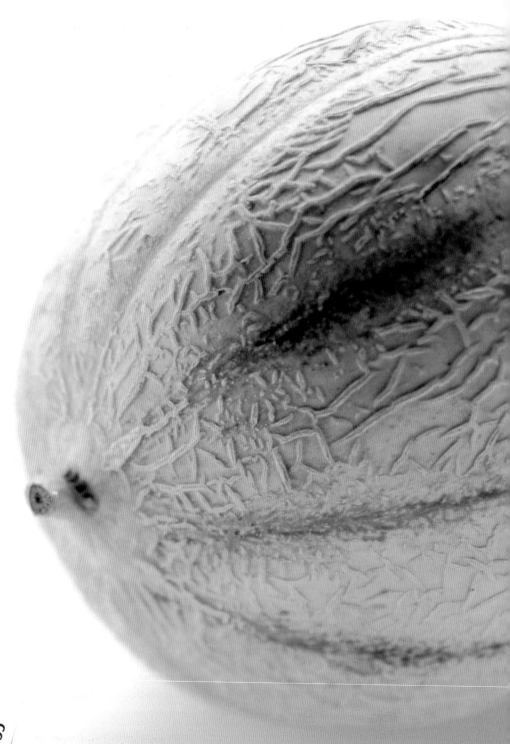

Yoghurt Drinks and Active Health Drinks

Of all the functional foods on the supermarket shelves, yoghurt drinks are amongst the most visible. While they claim to aid everything from bloating and tiredness to high cholesterol and digestive problems, the jury is still out on how effective some of these products are. If you do choose to buy them, pick yoghurts that are low in sugar and give precise information about the bacterial cultures they contain – and remember that even the best active drink is no substitute for a healthy diet.

PROBIOTICS AND PREBIOTICS

The chances are you have heard about "good" and "bad" bacteria from adverts for yoghurt drinks, but what do these terms really mean? The human intestine is full of bacteria, many of which – the "good" bacteria – live there naturally and are involved in the digestion of food. Others – the "bad" bacteria – can be potentially harmful. Prebiotic foods are those that help to encourage the growth of good bacteria in the gut by providing them with the nutrients they need. Examples include leeks, artichokes and bananas. Probiotics are foods (such as yoghurts) that are specially formulated to contain added live cultures of these good bacteria – the idea being that they will travel through the stomach and join the rest in the gut, helping the digestive system to work smoothly.

However, the Food Standards Agency published research from the University of Reading in March 2005, which showed that not all the strains of bacteria used in probiotic yoghurts survived the passage through the stomach to the intestines. It tested 11 different products and found that "overall, adding bacteria from probiotics did not change the total number of bacteria in the gut". This suggests that the effects of commercially available probiotics on digestive health may be limited.

There is some evidence that probiotics may be beneficial to people who suffer from gut infections, or whose bacteria count has been reduced as a result of diarrhoea.

HEALTH CLAIMS REGULATION

Despite the concerns of consumer bodies, adverts for probiotic yoghurts and active health drinks routinely give the impression that they might reinforce our immune systems (one brand, Actimel, uses the phrase "helps support your natural defences") – the implication being that people who don't fortify their diets may be more at risk of digestive problems. Some companies also claim that their products reduce stress, tiredness, bloating and a range of other complaints.

CHOLESTEROL-LOWERING DRINKS

Under the current voluntary scheme, the Joint Health Claims Initiative (www.jhci.co.uk) has approved a number of claims. These include the link between consumption of soya protein and reduced blood cholesterol, which may appear on the labels of some soya milk and yoghurt ~ducts. Another cholesterol claim, that plant sterols added to yoghurt drinks can lower blood cholesterol, has been widely researched and appears to be borne out in practice. Still, as the British Heart Foundation points out, "however effective plant sterols and stanols are proven to be, it is important to adopt a diet that is low in saturated fats with plenty of fruit and vegetables ... to stop smoking and to keep physically active".

Indeed, active and cholesterol-lowering drinks will be most beneficial if they are combined with a healthy diet. A good intake of fibre is crucial to digestive health, while low intakes of fats and saturates will have an impact on blood cholesterol. Yoghurt drinks are often high in sugar, so choose your brand carefully.

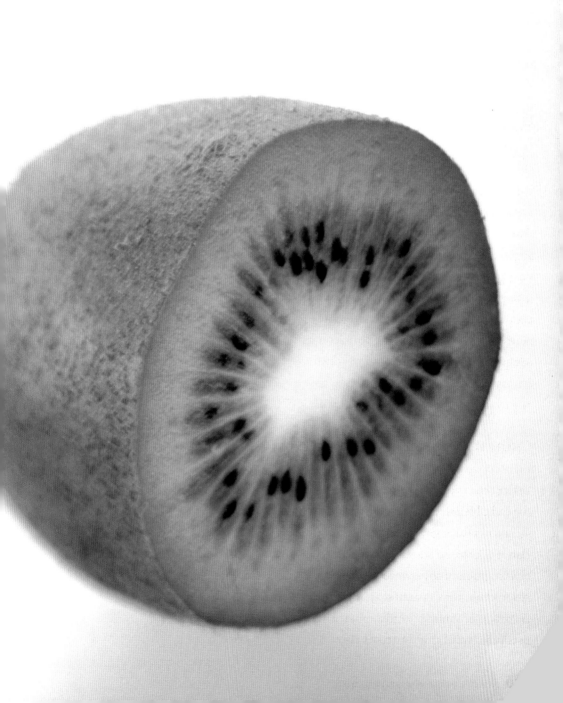

OUR RESEARCH RESULTS

Of the products included in the survey, Petits Filous Plus is the only one that doesn't claim any active properties. Flora Pro-activ and Benecol are both cholesterol-lowering drinks, while Yakult, Muller Vitality and Actimel all include pre- or probiotic bacteria for the digestive system. The Muller range also contains omega-3. Other than their functionality, the products appear very similar in their nutritional credentials: all are rated moderate for sugars and low for fats and saturated fat. None contain more than 0.3g of salt per 100g. Their calorie counts are also similar, with only Actimel 0.1% having significantly fewer calories at 28kcal per 100g, followed by Yakult Light with 473kcal per 100g.

As well as this, Actimel 0.1% and Yakult Light 47.3 are the only products to display a significant difference between the figures for carbohydrates and those for sugars. While it has 12.2g carbohydrates per 100g, only 7.3g of these are sugars. Benecol and Petits Filous Plus have the highest sugar levels, with 14.1g and 13.2g per 100g respectively. A check of the ingredients reveals that in many cases these figures will include added sugars such as glucose-fructose syrup. After Actimel 0.1%, Yakult has the lowest figure of 73g sugars. Interestingly, the Yakult product is the highest in fibre, at a full 1.8g per 100g. Actimel, Benecol and Petits Filous Plus contain none of this nutrient. They do, however, offer more protein than Yakult Light, with Actimel coming out highest at 3g per 100g. Flora Pro-activ contains the most fat, although the figure of 2.9g is still very low; Flora and Actimel also have the most saturates, at 1.1g per 100g. Unfortunately, the one thing these figures cannot show is how effective these products are as active supplements – that (for now) is a matter for personal experience.

THE GOOD NUTRITION GUIDE RECOMMENDS

LOWEST IN SUGARS:
Actimel 0.1%

LOWEST IN SATURATED FATS:
Actimel 0.1%

LOWEST IN SALT:
Benecol

YOGHURT DRINKS AND ACTIVE HEALTH DRINKS

BRAND NAME	ENERGY	PROTEIN	FIBRE	CARBOHYDRATES	SUGARS	FAT	SATURATED FAT	SALT	GOOD NUTRITION GUIDE SCORE	Company group
Actimel	72	3	0	10.5	10.5	1.6	1.1	0.1	87.5	Danone
Benecol	86	2.6	0	14.2	14.1	2.1	0.1	0.0	87.5	McNeil Nutritionals
Vitality 0.1% Red Berry	77	2.7	0.9	12.6	11.7	1.7	1.0	0.1	87.5	Muller's Dairy
Flora Pro-activ Strawberry	87	2.6	0.05	12.5	12.5	2.9	1.1	0.1	87.5	Unilever
Yakult Light	47.3	1.3	1.8	12.2	7.3	0.0	0.0	0.1	87.5	Yakult Honsha
Petits Filous Plus (Strawberry)	77	2.8	0	13.2	13.1	1.3	0.9	0.2	87.5	Yoplait
Actimel 0.1%	28	2.8	0	3.3	3.3	0.1	tr	0.1	100	Danone

Key

TYPICAL SERVING SIZE: 100g (one drink)

All figures are grammes per 100 grammes (expect Energy reading which = Kcal per100 grammes)

Source: The Ethical Company Organisation / The Good Nutrition Guide 2006 - 2008

For explantion of Good Nutrition Guide Score see the "Using the Research Tables" section

THE GOOD NUTRITION GUIDE
BEST CHOICE:

Actimel 0.1%

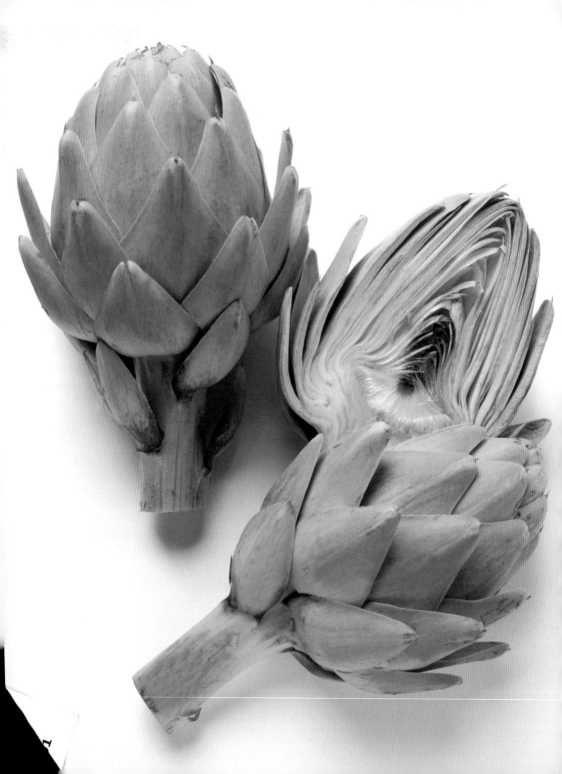

APPENDIX

RESOURCES •
BIBLIOGRAPHY •
ENDNOTES •

Resources

Nutritional information is based on public health advice from the Department of Health (www.dh.gov.uk), the NHS (www.nhs.uk), the Food Standards Agency (www.food.gov.uk) and the FSA's consumer website Eatwell (www.eatwell.gov.uk).

Non-governmental and industry sources include the British Nutrition Foundation (www.nutrition.org.uk), the Food Commission (www.foodcomm.org.uk) and consumer group Which? (www.which.co.uk).

The section on supermarkets draws on the work of Felicity Lawrence (author of Not On The Label) and Joanna Blythman (Shopped: The Shocking Power of British Supermarkets).

Bibliography

Joanna Blythman, Shopped: The Shocking Power of British Supermarkets (Harper Perennial, 2005)

Michael J Gibney, Hester H. Vorster and Frans J. Kok (eds.), Introduction to Human Nutrition (Blackwell, 2005)

Felicity Lawrence, Not On The Label (Penguin, 2004)

Peter Singer and Jim Mason, Eating: What We Eat and Why It Matters (Arrow Books, 2006)

Amanda Ursell, What Are You Really Eating? (Hay House, 2005)

GOVERNMENT, INDUSTRY AND INDEPENDENT BODIES

Advertising Standards Authority
www.asa.org.uk

British Cheese Board
www.cheeseboard.co.uk

British Nutrition Foundation
www.nutrition.org.uk

Department of Health
www.dh.gov.uk

Food Processing Technology
www.foodprocessing-technology.com

Food Standards Agency
www.food.gov.uk

Government News Network
www.gnn.gov.uk

Ice Cream Alliance
www.ice-cream.org

Institute of Food Research
www.ifr.ac.uk

Joint Health Claims Initiative
www.jhci.co.uk

National Health Service
www.nhs.uk

Ofcom
www.ofcom.org.uk

Office of Public Sector Information
www.opsi.gov.uk

PubMed
www.pubmed.gov

Soil Association
www.soilassociation.org

CAMPAIGNS, CONSUMER GROUPS AND CHARITABLE ORGANISATIONS

Allergy UK (British Allergy Foundation)
www.allergyuk.org

British Heart Foundation
www.bhf.org.uk

Diabetes UK
www.diabetes.org.uk

Eatwell (Food Standards Agency)
www.eatwell.gov.uk

5-a-day
www.5aday.nhs.uk

Food Commission
www.foodcomm.org.uk

Greenpeace
www.greenpeace.org.uk

My Pyramid
(United States Department of Agriculture)
www.mypyramid.gov

Salt (Food Standards Agency)
www.salt.gov.uk

Which?
www.which.co.uk

Vegan Society
www.vegansociety.com

Vegetarian Society
www.vegsoc.org